SAUNDERS MONOGRAPHS IN PHYSIOLOGY

CLINICAL GASTROINTESTINAL PHYSIOLOGY

D. NEIL GRANGER, Ph.D.

Professor, Department of Physiology,
College of Medicine, University of South Alabama,
Mobile, Alabama

JAMES A. BARROWMAN, M.D., Ph.D.

Professor, Faculty of Medicine and Assistant Dean of
Research and Graduate Studies, Memorial University
of Newfoundland, St. John's Newfoundland

PETER R. KVIETYS, Ph.D.

Associate Professor, Department of Physiology,
College of Medicine, University of South Alabama,
Mobile, Alabama

A SAUNDERS MONOGRAPH IN PHYSIOLOGY

1985

W. B. SAUNDERS COMPANY

*Philadelphia/London/Toronto/
Mexico City/Rio de Janeiro/Sydney/Tokyo*

W. B. Saunders Company: West Washington Square
Philadelphia, PA 19105

1 St. Anne's Road
Eastbourne, East Sussex BN21 3UN, England

1 Goldthorne Avenue
Toronto, Ontario M8Z 5T9, Canada

Apartado 26370—Cedro 512
Mexico 4, D.F., Mexico

Rua Coronel Cabrita, 8
Sao Cristovao Caixa Postal 21176
Rio de Janeiro, Brazil

9 Waltham Street
Artarmon, N.S.W. 2064, Australia

Ichibancho, Central Bldg., 22-1 Ichibancho
Chiyoda-Ku, Tokyo 102, Japan

Library of Congress Cataloging in Publication Data

Granger, D. Neil.
    Clinical gastrointestinal physiology.

    (Saunders monograph in physiology)
    1. Gastrointestinal system. 2. Gastroenterology.
I. Barrowman, J. A. II. Kvietys, Peter R. III. Title.
IV. Series. [DNLM: 1. Digestive System—physiology.
WI 102 G758c]
QP145.G68 1985   612′.32   84-26713
ISBN   0-7216-1283-0

Clinical Gastrointestinal Physiology   ISBN   0-7216-1283-0

Last digit is the print number: 9   8   7   6   5   4   3   2   1

For Cindy, Gwyn, and Kathy

PREFACE

The science of gastrointestinal physiology has expanded greatly during the past decade. A large part of the growth of knowledge of the digestive system stems from an increasing awareness of the impact of digestive diseases on modern medical practice. In spite of its importance, medical students are usually expected to devote relatively little time to the digestive system in their medical physiology course. Thus, there is a need for a textbook that is comprehensive yet concise and that allows the student to review the area of digestive system physiology within a two- to three-week time frame. This textbook was designed and written with this time frame in mind.

A unique organizational aspect of this book is the presentation of physiologic concepts with respect to the individual organs of the digestive system rather than the traditional classification into motor, absorptive, and secretory functions. Our approach allows the reader to follow a bolus of food down the gastrointestinal tract and learn the physiologic functions of the various organs that the bolus contacts either directly or indirectly (pancreas, liver). This approach serves to emphasize the sequential nature of the actions of each organ in the digestive system, and it places into perspective the contribution of each organ to the overall assimilation of a meal.

The first chapter introduces the reader to basic concepts pertaining to all or most organs in the digestive system. Chapters 2 through 8 review the major physiologic functions of the different organs comprising the digestive system. A similar format is used in these chapters in order to facilitate comparison of the functional characteristics of the various organs. In addition, a clinical correlation section is provided for each organ. The objective of the clinical correlations is to describe disorders of the digestive system that exemplify the importance of normal organ function. The final chapter describes the integrated response of the entire digestive system to a meal. Its objective is to provide the reader with an overview of how the individual organs interact in a concerted fashion to efficiently process a meal.

The authors are grateful to the many individuals who helped in the preparation of the manuscript. Our special thanks go to Sandy Worley for typing the entire manuscript, Penny Cook and Vicki Pitts for preparing the illustrations, and Drs. Patrick Tso and Joey Benoit for their critical appraisal of the text. We are also grateful for the support and encouragement of Drs. Aubrey E. Taylor and Albert R. Cox.

CONTENTS

ix

CLINICAL
GASTROINTESTINAL
PHYSIOLOGY

All organisms require energy for continued existence. This energy is derived from assimilation of chemical sources (nutrients) found in the environment. Single-celled organisms obtain these nutrients directly from the environment by simple processes such as diffusion and phagocytosis. By contrast, multicellular organisms have evolved a specialized system for assimilation of nutrients. In man, this system, the digestive system, takes the form of a tube, the internal surface of which constitutes an interface between the external environment and the circulatory system, which distributes the assimilated nutrients to all tissues of the body.

1

BASIC CONCEPTS

As shown in Figure 1–1, the gastrointestinal tract consists of the tube from mouth to anus (oropharynx, esophagus, stomach, small and large intestine) and associated secretory organs (salivary glands, liver, pancreas). Most of these components make a specialized contribution to the overall process of assimilation, i.e., digestion and absorption, while other components simply store or propel food. The mouth and esophagus are primarily involved in food propulsion. The stomach and colon are mainly involved in the storage of food and food residues, respectively. The salivary glands, pancreas, and liver manufacture and deliver digestive juices, while the primary site of digestion and absorption of food is the small intestine.

The medical significance of the digestive system is verified by the fact that a large proportion of patients consult their physicians concerning symptoms referable to the gastrointestinal tract. Common symptoms such as indigestion, nausea, vomiting, heartburn, abdominal discomfort, flatulence, constipation, and diarrhea frequently reflect disorders of function. Nevertheless, a significant proportion of these symptoms may indicate underlying disease processes. Gastrointestinal disorders translate into high medical costs (direct and due to disability) and many hours of diagnostic effort on the part of the physician. It is

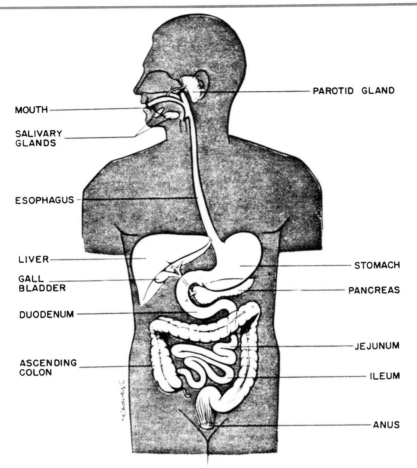

MOUTH

SALIVARY
GLANDS

ESOPHAGUS

LIVER

GALL
BLADDER

DUODENUM

ASCENDING
COLON

PAROTID GLAND

STOMACH

PANCREAS

JEJUNUM

ILEUM

ANUS

FIGURE 1–1. The digestive system. (From Guyton, A.C.: Textbook of Medical Physiology, 6th ed. Philadelphia, W.B. Saunders, 1981, p. 784.)

essential that the normal functions of the digestive system be understood before the physician can effectively treat these symptoms in a rational manner.

Current research is leading to a rapid expansion of our knowledge of the digestive system. This book provides the medical and graduate student with the fundamentals of gastrointestinal physiology. To illustrate the medical relevance of each area of gastrointestinal function, appropriate clinical correlations are made. The material in this text is presented using an organ approach, so that the reader can follow a bolus of food down the G.I. tract and learn physiologic functions of the various organs which the bolus contacts, either directly or indirectly. In order to minimize repetition of material, a brief summary of basic concepts is presented, which is essential to the understanding of the three major functions of the digestive system, i.e., motility, absorption, and secretion.

TABLE 1-1. Characteristics of the Major Gastrointestinal Hormones

Name	Composition	Local Stimuli for Release	Major Physiologic Action(s)	Circulating Half-life
Gastrin				
G17	peptide (2117 mw)	peptides, amino	acid secretion,	3 min
G34	peptide (3988 mw)	acids, distention	G.I. growth	12 min
Secretin	peptide (3056 mw)	duodenal acidity	pancreatic bicarbonate secretion	3 min
Cholecystokinin	peptide (3919 mw)	fatty acids amino acids	gallbladder contraction, pancreatic enzyme secretion and growth	5 min
Glucose-dependent insulinotropic peptide (GIP)	peptide (5105 mw)	glucose, fatty acids	insulin release	21 min

CONTROL OF GASTROINTESTINAL FUNCTION

Gastrointestinal Hormones and Peptides

It is now well recognized that a large number of hormones and related peptides are formed in tissues not generally regarded as part of the classic endocrine system. The gut and brain are examples of such tissues. Hormones are usually defined as chemical products of a tissue which are transported by the blood and have a specific regulatory effect upon target cells remote from their origin. Accordingly, there are cells scattered throughout the gut (mostly in the mucosa) which secrete peptides into the circulation to regulate important physiologic functions of the gastrointestinal tract. An example of such a substance is cholecystokinin (CCK), which is synthesized and released from the small intestinal mucosa in response to dietary fat. CCK reaches the gallbladder via the blood, causing it to contract and empty its contents (bile) into the gut lumen, thereby facilitating the process of fat absorption. In addition to CCK, there are three other peptides produced in the G.I. tract which meet all of the requirements for classification as a hormone, viz., secretin, gastrin, and glucose-dependent insulinotropic peptide (GIP) (Table 1-1).

There are several other peptides produced within the gastrointestinal tract which appear to have biologic activity, yet at present do not fulfill all of the requirements for hormone status. These substances are listed in Table 1-2. Some of the listed substances do not behave like classic hormones in that they are released from cells and diffuse through the extracellular space to their target cells. This type of local action is referred to as *paracrine* control. A good example of a paracrine agent is somatostatin, which exists throughout the gastrointestinal mucosa and pancreas at high concentrations and exerts local inhibitory action on gut endocrine cells. Peptides (vasoactive intestinal polypeptide) released from nerve terminals also fall under the broad category of paracrine agents, yet are specifically referred to as *neurocrines*.

TABLE 1–2. Peptides Produced in the Gastrointestinal Tract Having Biologic Activity but Not Fulfilling Requirements for Hormone Status

Vasoactive intestinal polypeptide
Motilin
Pancreatic polypeptide
Neurotensin
Somatostatin
Enteroglucagon
Substance P
Enkephalins
Villikinin
Enterogastrone
Thyrotropin releasing factor
Bulbogastrone
Urogastrone
Chymodenin
Entero-oxyntin

The technique of immunofluorescent histochemistry has allowed identification of the cells which produce specific gastrointestinal hormones, paracrines, and neurocrines. Although the individual cells are widely distributed, assays for peptide concentrations in gastrointestinal tissues reveal specific patterns of distribution as illustrated in Figure 1–2. The four established gastrointestinal hormones are found in highest concentrations in the upper gastrointestinal tract. On the other hand, neurotensin concentrations are highest in the distal portion of the G.I. tract.

It is now well recognized that the major physiologic stimuli for release of the four established gastrointestinal hormones are specific luminal constituents (Table 1–1). However, a significant portion of gastrin release is controlled by the vagus, with antral distention playing a minor role. How is the information regarding luminal composition transmitted to the endocrine cell? As a rule, endocrine cells in the mucosa have a small luminal surface with tufts of microvilli. The microvilli act as a receptor surface for sampling of luminal contents. Interaction of the luminal constituent with its receptor initiates the discharge of secretory granules located in the basal portion of the cell. Access of the hormone to the bloodstream is facilitated by the close proximity of the capillaries to the endocrine cell, and the fact that the capillary fenestrae (pores) always face the basal aspect of the cell. The time required for the hormone to diffuse across this short distance is only a few seconds.

The gastrointestinal hormones and most related peptides can be divided into two classes based upon the similarity of their amino acid sequence. One class consists of cholecystokinin and gastrin (Fig. 1–3A), which share an identical sequence of five amino acids at the carboxyterminal end of the chain. Since the two hormones share a common sequence of amino acids, they interact with the same receptor and thus exhibit similar actions. Nonetheless, the relative potency of action of the two hormones differs among target organs. This pre-

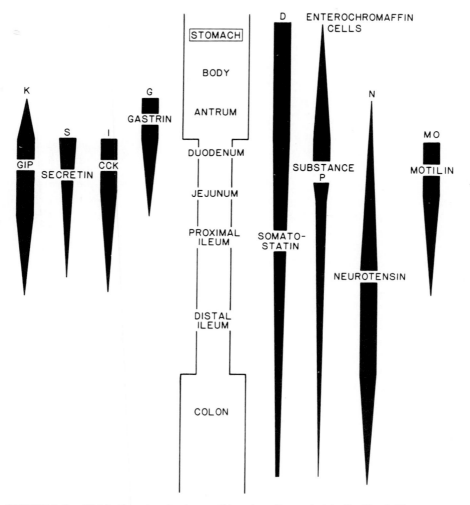

FIGURE 1–2.   Distribution of endocrine peptides along the gastrointestinal tract. The nomenclature of the cells of origin is indicated above each bar.

A. GASTRIN FAMILY

GASTRIN (17 AMINO ACIDS)

GLU-GLY-PRO-TRP-LEU-GLU-GLU-GLU-GLU-ALA-TYR-GLY-TRP-MET-ASP-PHE
SO_3H

CCK (33 AMINO ACIDS)

LYS-ALA-PRO-SER-GLY-ARG-VAL-SER-MET-ILE-LYS-ASN-LEU-GLN-SER-LEU-ASP-PRO-SER-HIS-ARG-ILE-SER-ASP-ARG-ASP-TYR-MET-GLY-TRP-MET-ASP-PHE
SO_3H

B. SECRETIN FAMILY

SECRETIN (27 AMINO ACIDS)

HIS-SER-ASP-GLY-THR-PHE-THR-SER-GLU-LEU-SER-ARG-LEU-ARG-ASP-SER-ALA-ARG-LEU-GLN-ARG-LEU-LEU-GLN-GLY-LEU-VAL

VIP (28 AMINO ACIDS)

" " " ALA-VAL- "   " ASP-ASN-TYR-THR- "   "   " LYS-GLN-MET-ALA-VAL-LYS-LYS-TYR- " ASN-SER-ILE-LEU-ASN

GIP (43 AMINO ACIDS)

" " " ILE- " ASP-TYR- " ILE-ALA-MET- " LYS-ILE- " GLN- " ASP-PHE-VAL-ASN-TRP- " LEU-ALA-GLN-14 MORE

GLUCAGON (29 AMINO ACIDS)

" " " " " " ASP-TYR- " LYS-TYR-LEU- " " ARG- " ALA- " ASP-PHE-VAL- " TRP- " MET-ASP-THR

FIGURE 1–3. The gastrin and secretin families of hormones. For the gastrin family the shared amino acid sequence is indicated by boxes. For the secretin family the amino acid residues identical to those in secretin are indicated by ("). (Adapted from Johnson, L.R.: Gastrointestinal Physiology. St. Louis, C.V. Mosby, 1981, pp. 4–5.)

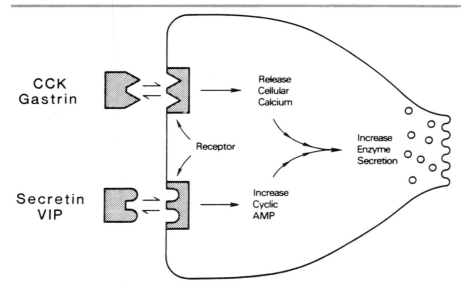

FIGURE 1–4. Intracellular mechanisms of hormone action. (Modified from Gardner, J.D., and Jensen, R.T. *In* Johnson, L.R. (ed.): Physiology of the Gastrointestinal Tract. New York, Raven Press, 1981, p. 834.)

sumably results from a difference in the receptors. For example, CCK is more potent than gastrin at receptors in gallbladder smooth muscle, while gastrin is more potent than CCK at receptors on the parietal cell of the stomach.

The second class of structurally similar peptides consists of secretin, vasoactive intestinal polypeptide (VIP), pancreatic glucagon, and GIP (Fig. 1–3B). There is no structural similarity between this class of hormones and the gastrin family. Unlike the gastrin family, the structural homologies are internal; i.e., identical amino acid sequences exist in segments within the peptide chain. The structural homologies within this group account for a shared spectrum of biologic activities. For example, the action of secretin and VIP on pancreatic duct cells is consistent with shared receptors.

Although the two classes of hormones are structurally dissimilar, the same effect in a target cell may result from hormones of either class. This is explained by the presence of receptors for each class on the same target cell. For example, in the pancreatic acini, the interaction of CCK or gastrin with their receptor leads to an increased intracellular Ca^{++} concentration, whereas the interaction of secretin and VIP with their receptor activates the cyclic AMP system (Fig. 1–4). Both of these "second messengers" (Ca^{++}, cyclic AMP) increase enzyme secretion by the cell. In contrast to other endocrine systems (e.g., pituitary-thyroid axis) in which feedback mechanisms exert fine control of hormone concentrations and actions, the secretion of gastrointestinal hormones is not subject to such fine control. Since the principal stimuli for release of G.I. hormones are the hydrolytic products of food, the blood concentrations of the hormones rise and fall in accordance with the passage of food through the G.I. tract. Nonetheless, it will become apparent that some degree of feedback control exists in the G.I. tract to optimize the efficiency of digestion and absorption.

Extrinsic and Intrinsic Nerves

The gastrointestinal tract is extensively innervated by both the sympathetic and parasympathetic divisions of the autonomic nervous system. Efferent fibers in the vagus (parasympathetic) and spinal (sympathetic) nerves allow the central nervous system to exert an influence on gastrointestinal function. Afferent fibers in these nerves carry information from G.I. organs to the brain. Furthermore, there is a complex intrinsic nervous system located within the wall of the stomach and gut. The intrinsic nervous system is perceived as an "enteric brain" which can function independently of the central nervous system to modulate the motor and secretory activities of the stomach and gut.

INTRINSIC INNERVATION

The intrinsic nervous system consists of two networks of ganglia and fibers located within the wall of the G.I. tract (Fig. 1–5) and extending from the esophagus to the anus. One network, the myenteric (Auerbach's) plexus, is situated between the circular and longitudinal muscle layers, while the submucosal (Meissner's) plexus separates the circular muscle and submucosal layers. Efferent fibers from the myenteric plexus terminate on smooth muscle cells in both the circular and longitudinal layers; therefore, this plexus primarily influences motility (muscle tone and rhythm). The submucosal plexus efferents terminate directly on the mucosal epithelium (including endocrine cells), on the muscularis mucosa, and, to some extent, on the circular muscle layer. Therefore, this plexus primarily influences epithelial cell activity (e.g., secretion) and to a lesser extent, motor functions. There are many short neurons linking the myenteric and submucosal plexuses. Afferent fibers from both plexuses relay sensory information (distention, pain) to the central nervous system.

EXTRINSIC INNERVATION

Parasympathetics

The parasympathetics have important secretomotor actions on the entire gastrointestinal tract. The organs of the digestive system are innervated by parasympathetic fibers originating from the medulla oblongata and the sacral part of the spinal cord (Fig. 1–6). The medullary outflow comprises the seventh, ninth, and tenth (vagus) cranial nerves. The fibers of the seventh and ninth nerves supply the salivary glands. The vagi supply fibers to the esophagus, stomach, small intestine, proximal part of the large bowel, pancreas, liver,

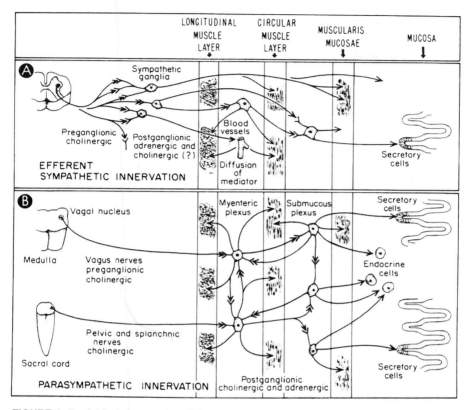

FIGURE 1–5. Intrinsic innervation of the gastrointestinal tract. *A*, Sympathetic innervation. *B*, Parasympathetic innervation. (From Davenport, H.W.: Physiology of the Digestive Tract. Chicago, Year Book Medical Publishers, 1977, p. 26.)

gallbladder, and bile ducts. The sacral parasympathetics originate from the second, third, and fourth sacral segments of the spinal cord and proceed to form the pelvic nerves (*nervi erigentes*). These fibers supply the distal portion of the large bowel, i.e., sigmoid, rectum, and anus.

The preganglionic neurons of the parasympathetic supply terminate primarily on the ganglionic cells of the myenteric plexus in the stomach and gut and on the intraparenchymal ganglion cells of the pancreas, salivary glands, and liver. The preganglionic neurotransmitter is acetylcholine, which interacts with *nicotinic* receptors on the postsynaptic membrane of ganglion cells. Acetylcholine also serves as a neurotransmitter at postganglionic nerve terminals, where it interacts with *muscarinic* receptors on effector cells (e.g., acinar cell of pancreas). Recently, a large number of putative postganglionic neurotransmitters have been identified. These include serotonin, purine nucleotides, vasoactive intestinal polypeptide, substance P, and the enkephalins.

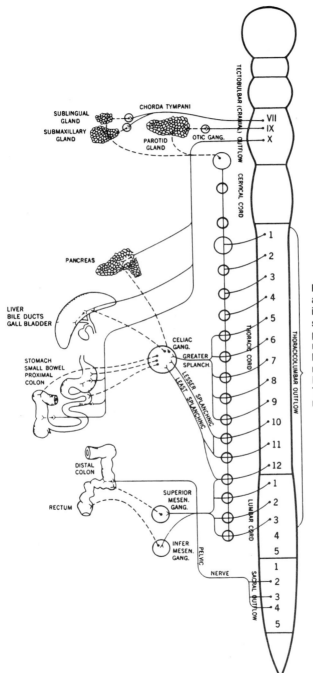

FIGURE 1–6. Extrinsic parasympathetic and sympathetic innervation of the digestive system. Solid lines represent preganglionic and broken lines represent postganglionic fibers. (Modified from Goodman, L.S., and Gilman, A.: The Pharmacological Basis of Therapeutics. New York, Macmillan Co., 1980.)

Sympathetics

Unlike the parasympathetic supply to the G.I. tract, which originates from the cranial and sacral segments of the cord, the sympathetic supply stems from the midportion of the cord, i.e., the thoracic and lumbar segments (Fig. 1–6). The preganglionic fibers enter the sympathetic chains after leaving the cord. The postganglionic fibers that terminate on the salivary glands arise directly from the superior cervical ganglia, which are located within the chains. All other digestive organs receive postganglionic fibers originating from outlying ganglia such as the celiac, superior mesenteric, and inferior mesenteric ganglia, which in turn receive preganglionic fibers from the sympathetic chain. The celiac ganglia supply fibers to the esophagus, stomach, proximal duodenum, liver, and pancreas; the superior mesenteric ganglia supply fibers to the remainder of the small bowel and proximal colon; and the inferior mesenteric ganglia supply fibers to the distal colon and rectum. Some fibers make synaptic connections with the intrinsic nerve plexuses of the stomach and gut, while others end directly on blood vessels and, to a lesser extent, on other parenchymal structures. Synaptic transmission between pre- and postganglionic fibers of the sympathetic nervous system involves acetylcholine, while the postganglionic neurotransmitter is norepinephrine.

Afferent Nerve Fibers

Afferent fibers from the G.I. tract also travel in autonomic nerves. For example, 80 per cent of vagal fibers and 50 per cent of the sympathetic fibers are afferent. All of these fibers transmit sensory information to the central nervous system. Some of this information reaches the conscious level, chiefly in the form of pain, while other information is a component of vegetative reflex arcs controlling gastrointestinal function. Sensations of pain emanating from the G.I. tract are carried in fibers whose cell bodies are located in the dorsal root ganglia. Afferent fibers involved in reflex regulation of G.I. functions form arcs which involve either the spinal cord, the celiac and mesenteric ganglia, or ganglia of the intrinsic nervous system. For example, the enterogastric reflex involves signals from sensory endings in the intestinal mucosa which pass along afferent fibers, whose cell bodies are located in the wall of the intestine (Fig. 1–7). These fibers synapse with cells in the celiac and mesenteric ganglia, which in turn send efferent fibers to the stomach wall. This reflex arc allows the intestine to influence the rate of gastric emptying.

GASTROINTESTINAL FUNCTIONS

Motility

Efficient assimilation of nutrients by the gastrointestinal tract depends on an orderly intraluminal flow of ingested food at a rate which allows for optimum

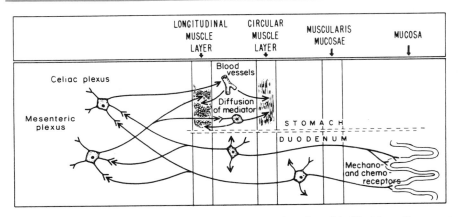

FIGURE 1–7.   Role of afferent fibers in the enterogastric reflex. (Modified from Davenport, H.W.: Physiology of the Digestive Tract. Chicago, Year Book Medical Publishers, 1977, p. 27.)

digestive and absorptive activity. Propulsion of food is accomplished by the coordinated motor activity of the gut—a function attributed to its smooth muscle coat. Not only is motility concerned with propulsive activity, but also with the mixing of foodstuff with digestive secretions. One important digestive secretion, bile, is delivered into the lumen of the gut by contraction of the smooth muscle lining the gallbladder.

The smooth muscle coat of the gut is characteristically arranged in two layers, an inner circular and an outer longitudinal. In addition, a thin layer of smooth muscle (the muscularis mucosa), whose function is not clearly understood, separates the mucosa from the submucosa. At the upper end of the gastrointestinal tract, striated muscle is found in the oropharynx and upper one third of the esophagus, and this striated muscle blends with the smooth muscle of the midesophagus. The remainder of the gastrointestinal tract is composed of smooth muscle except for the external anal sphincter, which consists of striated muscle. At various strategic points along the alimentary tract, specialized areas of smooth muscle serve to regulate the movement of chyme and secretions between adjacent luminal compartments. The term sphincter is applied to these regions, some of which are characterized by a thickened band of circular smooth muscle, e.g., the upper esophageal sphincter, the pylorus, and the sphincter of Oddi. Others are functional sphincters with no specialized structural features that generate a zone of high intraluminal pressure. The best example of these functional sphincters is the lower esophageal sphincter.

Gastrointestinal smooth muscle is characterized by a resting membrane potential which can depolarize, initiating contraction. The resting membrane potential of gastrointestinal smooth muscle (as measured with microelectrodes) ranges from -55 mv to -80 mv, with a mean of about -60 mv. This potential is created by the distribution of Na^+, K^+, and Cl^- ions across the cell membrane. Their relative distribution is governed by three factors: the membrane conductance for each ion species, the Donnan effect, and the Na^+-K^+ pump.

The conductance for each ion across a given membrane will determine the distribution of charge across that membrane. At equilibrium, the potential generated across the membrane for a given ion can be expressed mathematically in the terms of the Nernst equation

$$E_m \text{ (millivolts)} = \pm\ 61 \log C_1/C_2$$

where E_m is the equilibrium potential across the membrane, and C_1 and C_2 represent the concentrations of the ions in the two compartments separated by the membrane. In addition to the conductance of the membrane to different ion species, the Donnan effect can influence the distribution of ionic charge across the membrane of cells by limiting the diffusion of negatively charged intracellular proteins. These forces are a result of the simple physical laws governing diffusion of ions. Most cell membranes also possess a Na^+-K^+ pump, which actively extrudes sodium and recovers potassium (Na^+,K^+-ATPase). Since the pump moves a larger number of sodium ions out than potassium ions in (3 Na^+ to 2 K^+), it causes a net transfer of positive charge out of the cell and thus contributes to the resting membrane potential. When the values for the relative conductance and equilibrium potentials for Na^+, K^+, and Cl^- in smooth muscle are used to calculate the resting membrane potential, a value of approximately -40 mv is obtained. The additional 20 mv of the observed membrane potential is generally attributed to the electrogenic Na^+-K^+ pump.

In contrast to most other excitable tissues, where the resting membrane potential remains fairly constant, the resting potential of gastrointestinal smooth muscle is characterized by rhythmic fluctuations (Fig. 1–8). The oscillations of the potential have an amplitude of 15 to 20 mv, a duration of 1 to 5 sec, and a frequency which varies along the gut, i.e., 3/min in the stomach, 12/min in the duodenum, declining progressively to 9/min in the ileum. These rhythmic depolarizations have been termed slow waves or the *basal electrical rhythm.* Slow waves seem to be due to fluctuations in the activity of the Na^+-K^+ pump, since they disappear with the application of ouabain to smooth muscle. However, cyclic changes in membrane conductance to diffusible ions (e.g., Na^+ or Cl^-) may also be involved.

Superimposed on the depolarization phase of the slow wave are small generator potentials, which, when they reach a critical threshold voltage, give rise to a spike or action potential (Fig. 1–8). It is these spikes that are responsible for initiating muscle contraction, the strength of the contraction being determined by the number of spikes generated. The prepotential and action potential involve an influx of Na^+ or Ca^{++} into the smooth muscle cell, owing to changes in membrane conductance for these ions. The Ca^{++} entering the cell is intimately involved in the initiation of smooth muscle contraction.

The contractile activity of smooth muscle can be compared to and contrasted with that of striated muscle. Smooth muscle cells are much smaller and

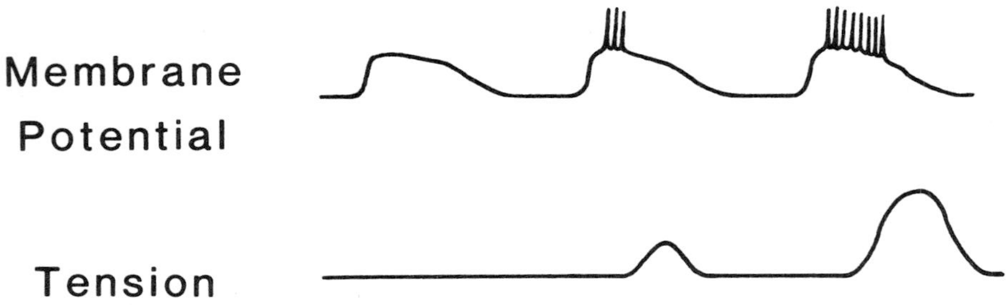

Membrane
Potential

Tension

FIGURE 1–8. Relationship between slow waves, spike activity, and generation of tension in intestinal smooth muscle. Note that smooth muscle contraction (increased tension) occurs only when spike potentials are present on the slow waves. The strength of the contraction is directly related to the number of spikes. (Modified from Cohen, S., and Snape, W.J. *In* Sleisenger, M.H., and Fordtran, J.S. (eds.): Gastrointestinal Disease: Pathophysiology, Diagnosis, Management. 3rd ed. Philadelphia, W.B. Saunders, 1983, p. 859.)

have a greater surface-to-volume ratio than have skeletal muscle cells. Although both muscle types contain similar contractile proteins (actin and myosin filaments) that require Ca^{++} for activation, the excitation-contraction coupling is somewhat different in smooth and striated muscle cells. The rise in intracellular Ca^{++} in smooth muscle is primarily a result of an influx of extracellular Ca^{++}, whereas mobilization of intracellular stores is more important in striated muscle. The high surface-to-volume ratio in smooth muscle cells facilitates the influx and intracellular diffusion of calcium. Smooth muscle cells lack troponin, which is present in skeletal muscle cells. Therefore, it is thought that Ca^{++} initiates smooth muscle contraction via calmodulin-mediated activation of myosin filaments. As in striated muscle, the energy for contraction is derived from degradation of ATP.

Smooth muscle contraction does not begin until 50 to 100 milliseconds after excitation and requires an additional 500 milliseconds for development of maximum tension. The entire cycle requires 1 to 3 seconds and is 30 times longer than a single twitch contraction of skeletal muscle. The latency to onset of contraction is due to the time required for Ca^{++} to enter and diffuse throughout the cell. The slow relaxation depends on the removal of Ca^{++} by intracellular depots.

How is electrical and contractile activity propagated longitudinally and perpendicularly in the two layers of the gastrointestinal tract? A fundamental feature of smooth muscle cells is the presence of *gap junctions* or *nexi*, which confer the properties of a functional syncytium. These gap junctions provide a low resistance pathway for the movement of ions and thereby facilitate electrical conduction from cell to cell. Although prevalent in circular smooth muscle, they are sparse in longitudinal muscle; thus other mechanisms for the spread of electrical and contractile activity within this layer must exist. Coupling be-

Motility pattern	Site	Function

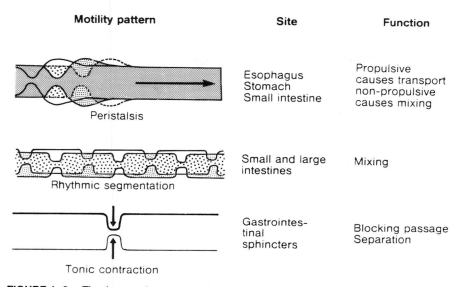

Peristalsis — Esophagus, Stomach, Small intestine — Propulsive causes transport non-propulsive causes mixing

Rhythmic segmentation — Small and large intestines — Mixing

Tonic contraction — Gastrointestinal sphincters — Blocking passage Separation

FIGURE 1–9. The three major patterns of gastrointestinal motility. (Modified from Waldeck, F. *In* Schmidt, R.F., and Thews, G. (eds.): Human Physiology. Berlin, Springer-Verlag, 1983, p. 588.)

tween the longitudinal and circular smooth muscle layers also exists, as evidenced by the lack of slow waves in isolated circular muscle as compared with isolated longitudinal muscle. However, slow waves can be detected in both layers in the intact system. The means of this electrical coupling is not clear; however, possible links include the myenteric plexus or connective tissue bridges.

Electrical and contractile events in gastrointestinal smooth muscle lead to three major patterns of motility: rhythmic segmentation, peristalsis, and tonic contractions (Fig. 1–9). Rhythmic segmentation, which is attributed to the activity of the circular muscle layer, mixes ingested nutrients with digestive secretions. In addition, segmentation tends to move intestinal contents analward, because the frequency of contractions is higher in the upper than lower small intestine. Another contributory factor to forward propulsion of luminal content is peristaltic activity along the gastrointestinal tract. Peristaltic contractions consist of a wave of circular muscle contraction which propels lumen contents in an aboral direction. The contractile wave is coupled to a wave of relaxation in the adjacent downstream section of the bowel. Although peristalsis can be conducted in both directions, reflex relaxation, an event mediated by the myenteric plexus, is believed to confer the observed polarity on peristaltic activity, i.e., in an analward direction.

Tonic contraction, with intermittent relaxation, of the sphincters serves to regulate the movement of luminal contents. Relaxation of these sphincters is mediated by reflexes involving the myenteric plexus. Receptive relaxation is another feature of gastrointestinal organs (notably the stomach) attributed, in part, to the response of smooth muscle to stretch. When a segment of smooth muscle is stretched to twice its original length, the tension generated is quickly dissipated. This phenomenon, termed stress-relaxation, is made possible by the loose arrangement of the actin and myosin filaments in smooth muscle cells.

Contractile activity of the gastrointestinal tract is regulated by both intrinsic and extrinsic influences on the basal electrical rhythm. For example, the post-ganglionic parasympathetic (vagus) neurotransmitter, acetylcholine, reduces the overall membrane potential while preserving the basal electrical rhythm, thereby increasing the tendency for spike discharge and contractile activity. Catecholamines, on the other hand, tend to hyperpolarize or stabilize the membrane against other agents that cause depolarization. In general, sympathetic discharge tends to reduce gastrointestinal motor activity, while parasympathetic discharge enhances it. In addition to these classic neurotransmitters, substances such as secretin, gastrin, cholecystokinin, insulin, and glucagon exert effects on gastrointestinal motility. Gastrin, CCK, and insulin tend to stimulate contractions, while secretin and glucagon depress motor activity.

Digestion

The human diet consists largely of carbohydrate, protein, and fat derived from animal and vegetable sources. These chemically complex substances are reduced to smaller absorbable units by digestive enzymes. The chemical reaction catalyzed by these enzymes is hydrolysis, which occurs primarily in the small intestine. Hydrolysis can occur within the gut lumen, at the apical membrane of the absorptive cell, or within the cytoplasm of this cell, depending on the location of the digestive enzymes. Intraluminal hydrolysis, the initial digestive event, is accomplished primarily by enzymes secreted by the glands associated with the gastrointestinal tract, of which the pancreas is the most important. All three classes of nutrients must undergo preliminary hydrolysis in the lumen in order for effective absorption to occur. In the case of fat, this digestive step is facilitated by biliary secretions and yields monoglycerides and fatty acids, which require no further modification before absorption. Proteins and carbohydrates, on the other hand, undergo further processing. Intraluminal hydrolysis reduces the glucose polymers (starch and glycogen) to a mixture of mono- and oligosaccharides, containing up to 4 to 5 glucose units. The oligosaccharides are further hydrolyzed to yield glucose moieties by saccharidases located in the apical membrane of mucosal cells. Intraluminal hydrolysis of proteins also yields a mixture of smaller fragments consisting of amino acids and oligomers of amino acids, such as di- and tripeptides. The peptides are further processed by peptidases, located in both the apical membrane and cytoplasm of the absorptive cells, to yield amino acids.

The sources of intraluminal digestive enzymes are the digestive glands,

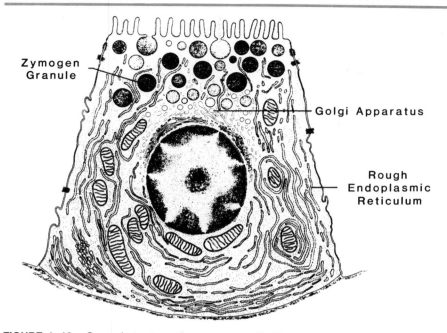

Zymogen Granule

Golgi Apparatus

Rough Endoplasmic Reticulum

FIGURE 1–10. General structure of a secretory cell. (From Ito, S. *In* Johnson, L.R. (ed.): Physiology of the Gastrointestinal Tract. New York, Raven Press, 1981, p. 539.)

some of which are located in the digestive tract itself (e.g., gastric glands), while others lie outside the alimentary tract (pancreas and salivary glands) and deliver their secretions to the gut lumen through ducts. Figure 1–10 illustrates schematically the general structure of a secretory cell. Digestive enzymes are proteins and are synthesized, stored, and secreted by these specialized cells. The secretion of proteins (i.e., enzymes) is an orderly process, beginning with synthesis of the peptide chain in the basal portion of the cell and culminating with extrusion of the proteins at the apical region. The secretory cycle can be divided into the following six intracellular events: synthesis, segregation, intracellular transport, concentration, storage, and discharge. The enzymes are synthesized by polysomes attached to the rough endoplasmic reticulum, and the elongating peptide chain is directed into the cavity (cisterna) of the endoplasmic reticulum. This form of synthesis effectively segregates the secretory proteins to a membrane-bound compartment, which assures appropriate channeling of the protein through a series of subcellular organelles to their ultimate site of secretion. The newly synthesized proteins move through the cisternae to "transitional elements" of the rough endoplasmic reticulum that are subsequently pinched off and transport the proteins to the concentrating vacuoles of the Golgi apparatus. Within these vacuoles, the nascent proteins are concentrated to produce mature storage granules (zymogen granules). After their formation in the Golgi complex, the secretory granules migrate to the apical portion of the cell and remain there until an appropriate stimulus (neural or humoral) triggers exocytosis. Exocytosis involves the orderly movement of the granule toward the apical cell membrane and fusion of the zymogen granule and cell membrane. Then the membranes dissolve at the point of fusion, releasing the granule contents from the cell.

Absorption

Absorption in the gastrointestinal tract involves the uptake of a heterogeneous group of substances (water, electrolytes, and nutrients) from an aqueous medium. These substances vary in several important aspects which determine their mode of absorption, such as molecular size, charge (or lack thereof), and their relative aqueous and lipid solubilities.

ROUTES OF ABSORPTION

Solutes encounter various barriers and channels during their transit from the bulk aqueous phase of luminal content to the blood and lymphatic circulations during the process of absorption. The first barrier is the unstirred water layer lying adjacent to the luminal surface of the cell membrane. This layer is estimated to be 0.5 to 1 mm thick and hinders the diffusion of nutrients, particularly lipids, from the bulk aqueous phase to the membrane of the absorptive cell. The next barrier is the cell membrane and its associated structures. The cell membrane, a lipid bilayer containing phospholipids and cholesterol, has a mosaic pattern of proteins and glycoproteins associated with it. The glycocalyx consists of glycoprotein molecules and occurs on the luminal surface of the membrane (Fig. 1–11). Its function is not clearly understood at present, but it may serve as an attachment site for extrinsic hydrolytic enzymes such as pancreatic hydrolases.

The proteins of the cell membrane can be classified as either integral or peripheral. Integral proteins are embedded in the phospholipid bilayer, bridging it from its extracellular to intracellular surface. The peripheral proteins are attached to either surface and are believed to subserve primarily enzymatic functions. The integral proteins behave as enzymes or carriers and provide structural channels through the lipid membrane. The large surface area offered by the exposed lipid portion of the membrane allows for easy passive transit of lipid-soluble molecules into the cell, regardless of their size. For water and water-soluble molecules, the lipid membrane provides a more formidable barrier to entry into the cell; therefore, they utilize the structural proteins to traverse the cell membrane. Aqueous channels formed by the integral proteins provide a route of access to the cell interior for small water-soluble substances such as electrolytes and water. The dimensions of these channels (or pores) in gastrointestinal epithelia average about 8 Å in diameter, with larger pores in the duodenum than in the ileum. Since these channels are created by charged proteins, electrolyte movement through them may be either facilitated or hindered, depending on the ion species and the pore charge. For example, the epithelium of the gallbladder has an excess of negatively charged pores, while in the stomach cationic pores predominate.

Another route by which electrolytes and water cross the mucosal epithelia is via the tight junctions connecting adjacent absorptive cells (Fig. 1–11). These paracellular or intercellular channels behave as if they have different degrees of porosity in different tissues. For example, much more fluid and electrolytes cross the intercellular junctions of the gallbladder epithelium than cross the intestinal epithelium.

Neither the tight junctions nor the protein channels of the cell membrane offer suitable routes for the absorption of large water-soluble nutrients such as glucose and amino acids. For the uptake of these substances, mechanisms exist that involve specialized "carrier" proteins. These proteins can "shuttle" molecules across the cell membrane. For large molecules, the possibility also exists that pinocytosis may account for cellular uptake from the intestinal lumen. The quantitative significance of this possibility is not clear at present but is probably slight.

The remaining barriers in the absorptive process are the basolateral membrane of the enterocyte, its basement membrane, the interstitium of the lamina propria, and the endothelial cell wall of capillaries and lymphatics. Relatively little is known about these barriers. Located in the basolateral cell membrane are energy-dependent ion pumps which promote the exit of electrolytes and water. Larger water-soluble molecules, such as monosaccharides and amino acids, appear to diffuse across the membrane. Chylomicrons (750 to 6000 Å in diameter), which are formed in the cell during fat absorption, leave by exocytosis through the basolateral cell membrane. The lateral intercellular space between enterocytes (Fig. 1–11) is the final common pathway for a heterogeneous collection of water, solutes, and lipid particles which then cross the basement membrane, traverse the interstitium, and reach the blood and lymphatic circulations. The water-soluble substances enter blood capillaries, and particulate lipids enter the initial lymphatics.

MECHANISMS OF ABSORPTION

Substances are absorbed by two basic processes, diffusion and active transport. Diffusion can be defined as the movement of molecules along a concentration or electrical gradient or both. Diffusion is a passive process governed by simple physical laws and requires no energy input. Active transport, on the other hand, involves the movement of molecules uphill against a concentration, electrical, or pressure gradient and therefore requires energy.

Passive Absorption

Lipid-soluble substances cross the lipid portion of the cell membrane in accordance with their concentration gradient. Water-soluble substances can

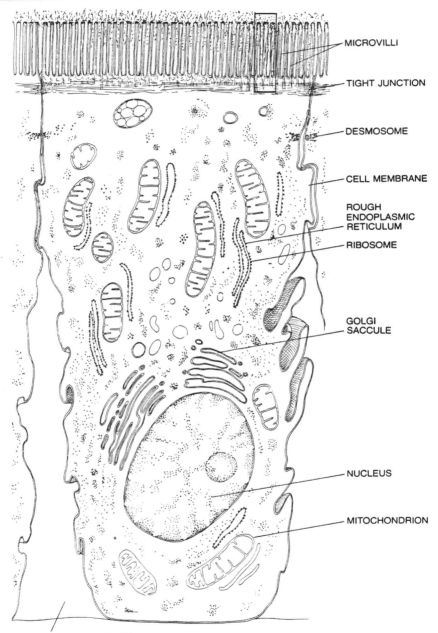

FIGURE 1–11.   General structure of an absorptive cell. (From Moog, F.: The lining of the small intestine. Sci. Am., *245*:160, 1981.)

Illustration continues on the opposite page

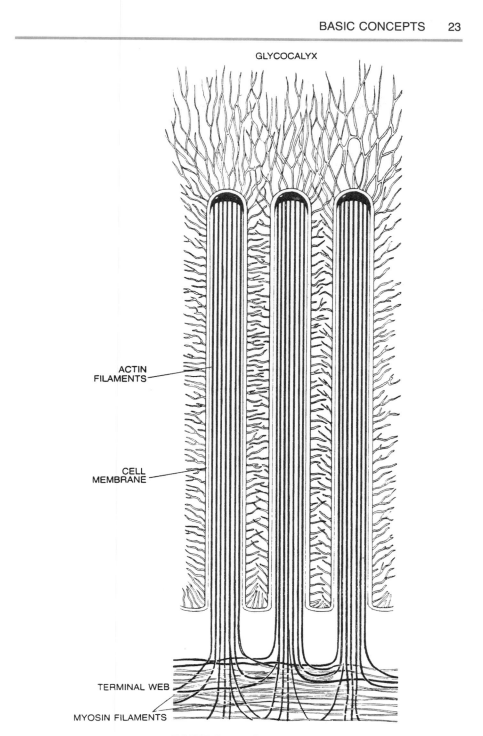

FIGURE 1–11. *Continued*

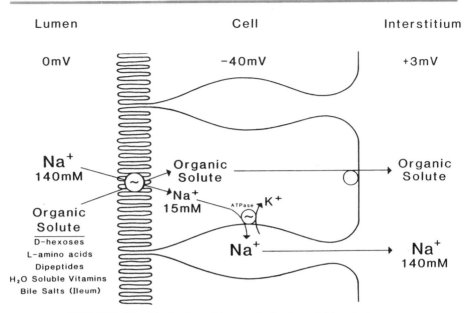

FIGURE 1–12. Mechanism of transport of water-soluble substances.

also enter the cell by passive diffusion. Small solutes (electrolytes), whose dimensions are smaller than the aqueous pores, can diffuse through these channels. Larger water-soluble molecules are obliged to use an alternative route involving carrier proteins in the membrane (Fig. 1–12). The molecule to be transported, such as the monosaccharide fructose, couples with its carrier on the external side of the membrane and the complex either diffuses or rotates within the membrane. At the inner face of the membrane the transported molecule dissociates from its carrier. This carrier is analogous to the aqueous pores in that the laws governing simple diffusion still operate, and this process is termed *facilitated diffusion*. However, an important difference exists between simple diffusion and facilitated diffusion. Since facilitated diffusion depends on a fixed number of carrier protein sites, this process is saturable, unlike simple diffusion.

Active Absorption

Water-soluble substances can also be actively transported across the cell membrane. Actively transported substances include ions such as Na^+, K^+, Cl^-, H^+, Ca^{++}, and Fe^{++}, as well as certain monosaccharides, amino acids, and peptides. Active transport processes can be divided into two main types, primary and secondary (electrolyte-coupled).

An example of a primary active transport process is the exchange of Na^+

and K^+ across the cell membrane as illustrated in Figure 1–12. The active transport of Na^+ and K^+ is a characteristic of all cells in the body and is responsible for the extracellular and intracellular distribution of these ions. Both ions are moved against their concentration gradients by means of a carrier protein possessing enzymatic activity (Na^+, K^+-ATPase). The enzymatic activity of this carrier provides the energy required for transport by virtue of its intrinsic ability to hydrolyze ATP. The hydrolysis of ATP occurs on the inner portion of the membrane, and the energy so derived enables the carrier to transport sodium out of the cell and potassium into the cell. The transport of these ions is coupled in such a manner that three Na^+ ions are extruded for every two K^+ ions taken in. In the absorptive epithelia of both the intestine and gall-bladder, the Na^+-K^+ pump is located in the basolateral portion of the cells.

Secondary, or electrolyte-coupled transport, is a very important mechanism for the active absorption of monosaccharides, amino acids, and peptides. An example of electrolyte-coupled transport is the absorption of glucose by the enterocyte (Fig. 1–12). As mentioned above, the sodium-potassium pump is located in the basolateral portion of the epithelial cell and, by depleting intracellular sodium, it increases the concentration gradient for the diffusion of Na^+ from the lumen into the mucosal cell. The apical portion of the cell membrane contains a Na^+-solute (e.g., glucose) carrier protein. The carrier has binding sites for both glucose and Na^+, and it will not traverse the membrane unless both Na^+ and glucose are attached. Glucose and Na^+ are moved into the apical portion of the enterocyte by facilitated diffusion down a Na^+ concentration gradient created by the energy-dependent Na^+-K^+ pump in the basolateral membrane. This mechanism can transport glucose against its concentration gradient when necessary, that is, when intraluminal concentrations of glucose are low compared to intracellular levels. The glucose then leaves the basolateral portion of the cell and moves down its concentration gradient by facilitated diffusion. Thus, the overall movement of glucose from the intestinal lumen to the circulation is an active process deriving its energy from the Na^+-K^+ pump. A similar electrolyte-coupled transport mechanism is also important for the active absorption of other water-soluble nutrients such as amino acids and peptides.

WATER ABSORPTION

The absorption of water occupies a special position in gastrointestinal physiology in that up to 10 liters of water are normally transported from the lumen to the blood every 24 hours. How is this water absorbed? Water transport is accomplished by osmotic forces generated by solute absorption as described above. The "standing osmotic gradient" theory for water absorption across epithelial sheets was developed from studies on gallbladder epithelium (Fig. 1–13). According to the original hypothesis, a standing osmotic gradient is generated by active transport of sodium from the cell in the upper portion of the basolateral membrane just adjacent to the tight junction. The tight junction

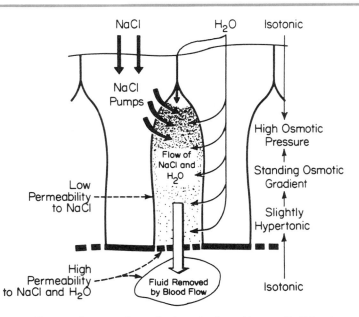

FIGURE 1–13. The standing osmotic gradient mechanism of transepithelial water movement. (Modified from Davenport, H.W.: Physiology of the Digestive Tract. Chicago, Year Book Medical Publishers, 1977, p. 155.)

itself was regarded as impermeable to water and electrolytes, and the hypertonicity in the lateral intercellular space drew water, by osmosis, from the lumen through the cell and into this space. The accumulation of fluid would lead to a rise in hydrostatic pressure in this compartment and drive the fluid into the absorbing blood and lymphatic vessels in the lamina propria of the mucosa. Although the basic principles of this concept still hold, recent revisions have been necessary to accommodate the fact that tight junctions and the cell membrane are more permeable to water and electrolytes than previously assumed. The revised version of the osmotic gradient theory predicts that a smaller osmotic pressure gradient will be created and does not require that sodium pumping be limited to a specific region of the membrane (Fig. 1–13). In view of the greater membrane permeabilities, it is predicted that the osmotic pressure differences required to drive water absorption are smaller than previously thought and need not exceed 3 to 5 mOsm/liter. This model allows for water absorption by both transcellular and paracellular routes. When large volumes of water are moved by osmotic gradients developed during solute absorption, the phenomenon of solvent drag (convection) is observed. This solvent drag results in the movement of a proportion of solutes against their electrical and chemical gradients.

SECRETION OF WATER AND ELECTROLYTES

Approximately 80 per cent of the water and electrolytes that are absorbed by the mucosal epithelium of the small and large bowel were originally secreted by the gut and its associated glands. Electrolyte secretion by gastrointestinal epithelium involves mechanisms comparable to those described earlier for absorption, the major difference being the direction of solute transport, i.e., lumen-to-blood movement with absorption and blood-to-lumen movement with secretion. As with absorption, an osmotic gradient is established by electrolyte secretion; therefore, water movement also occurs in the direction of blood to lumen.

CIRCULATION OF THE DIGESTIVE SYSTEM

The digestive organs receive the largest fraction of cardiac output, i.e., 25 to 30 per cent. This high rate of perfusion is presumably required to meet the metabolic needs of this large mass of tissue. Following a meal, blood flow to all digestive organs increases to meet the enhanced demand imposed by absorption and secretion. Inasmuch as the processes of absorption and secretion involve the transport of large volumes of fluid and solutes between the blood and gut lumen, the circulation plays an important role in these processes.

The organization of the blood supply to the gastrointestinal tract can be characterized in terms of parallel and series coupled circuits. The three major arteries supplying the digestive organs are the celiac, superior mesenteric, and inferior mesenteric arteries (Fig. 1–14). These vessels compose the parallel vascular circuit. The venous drainage from the stomach, pancreas, and intestines empties into the portal vein which, in turn, perfuses the liver and constitutes the series component of this circuit. The parallel arrangement of the splanchnic circulation allows for independent regulation of blood flow to individual organs in the G.I. tract, while the series arrangement of the portal venous system ensures that the liver is exposed to all absorbed substances.

There are several characteristic features of the microcirculation of digestive organs that optimize the ability of these tissues to move large amounts of fluid and electrolytes between the blood and transporting epithelia. In comparison to other tissues (e.g., skeletal muscle), the digestive organs have a high capillary density and consequently a large capillary surface area for secretion or absorption. The capillaries in the digestive organs are generally of the fenestrated type. These fenestrations provide an enormous pore area for water and solute exchange. Furthermore, the fenestrations usually face the basal aspect of the transporting cell, thereby minimizing the distance fluid must travel between

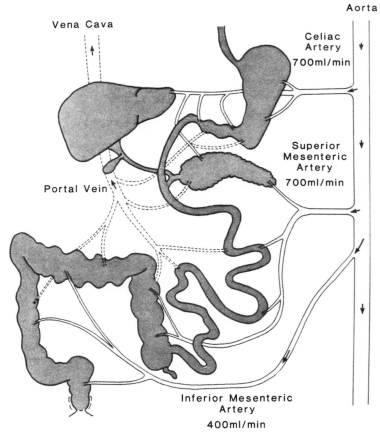

FIGURE 1–14.   The splanchnic circulation.

the blood and epithelia. Capillaries of digestive organs are highly permeable to small solutes, yet they are relatively impermeable to macromolecules. This means that molecules the size of glucose readily gain access to the blood stream, while plasma proteins are highly restricted by the capillary wall.

The lymphatic system also plays an important role in the transport functions of digestive organs. Lymphatic vessels are particularly prominent in the small bowel. Although blood flow is about 1000 times greater than lymph flow in digestive organs, approximately 1 to 2 liters of thoracic duct lymph is derived from the G.I. tract in man every 24 hours, and this lymph is the major route of fat transport to the circulation.

The amount of food and water ingested by a person is determined principally by the drives of hunger and thirst. These drives assure that the intake of food and water is appropriate for the needs of the individual. Following food and fluid ingestion, initial events in the mouth, such as mastication and salivation, prepare the food bolus for swallowing. This chapter describes these early events in food assimilation, which are collectively referred to as eating.

2

EATING: SALIVATION, MASTICATION, AND DEGLUTITION

PHYSIOLOGY OF HUNGER AND THIRST

Hunger

Hunger is defined as a craving for food. It is associated with a series of objective sensations such as hunger pangs. Accompanying phenomena include salivation and increased food-searching behavior. The term appetite is often used in the same sense as hunger; however, it more aptly describes attitudes toward different types of food. Appetite may persist even when hunger has been appeased. Satiety is the lack of a desire to eat that occurs after ingestion

31

of food. Anorexia, on the other hand, is an aversion to eating despite an existing stimulus for hunger.

Regulation of food intake occurs primarily within hypothalamic centers (Fig. 2–1). Hypothalamic regulation of feeding involves the interaction of two groups of nuclei referred to as the "satiety center" and the "feeding center." The satiety center is localized in the ventromedial nucleus, while the feeding center is situated in the ventrolateral nucleus. Stimulation of the ventrolateral nucleus evokes eating behavior in conscious animals, and its destruction causes severe fatal anorexia. On the other hand, stimulation of the ventromedial nucleus causes cessation of eating, while lesions in this region lead to excessive eating (hyperphagia). There is evidence indicating that these two centers interact in a reciprocal manner to regulate the desire for food. The feeding center is tonically active and is intermittently inhibited by the satiety center, i.e., following a meal.

Several factors are known to influence the hypothalamic centers controlling food intake. These include the primary nutrients (glucose, fats, amino acids), afferent nerve fibers from the stomach, temperature, gastrointestinal hormones, and neural influences from higher centers. An example of nutrient control of food intake is the "glucostat theory," which states that the glucose receptors present in the ventromedial nucleus of the hypothalamus are sensitive to changes in blood glucose levels. The hyperglycemia associated with feeding activates the satiety center and consequently inhibits feeding. Hypoglycemia has the opposite effect.

Gastric distention after a meal elicits afferent nervous signals to the hypothalamus which inhibit further feeding. Following food intake, metabolism of nutrients leads to a rise in body heat production (specific dynamic action of food). There are centers in the hypothalamus which are sensitive to temperature. The rise in body temperature after feeding leads to a suppression of the feeding center. Cholecystokinin, which is released during digestion, has been shown to suppress feeding in experimental animals. It is also well known that emotional disturbances affect eating patterns, presumably through neural connections between higher centers and the hypothalamus.

Thirst

Fluid intake is also controlled by a specific region of the hypothalamus called the thirst center (Fig. 2–2). This center is located anterior to the supraoptic nuclei in the lateral preoptic area of the hypothalamus. Stimulation of this area results in drinking. The thirst center is activated by increased extracellular fluid osmolality and decreased extracellular fluid volume. Injection of a hypertonic solution into the thirst center causes cell shrinkage which, in turn, stimulates thirst. This observation suggests that cells of the thirst center act as osmoreceptors, which control thirst and drinking. Reductions in extracellular fluid volume stimulate thirst through a mechanism independent of the osmoreceptor system. The renin-angiotensin system has been implicated in

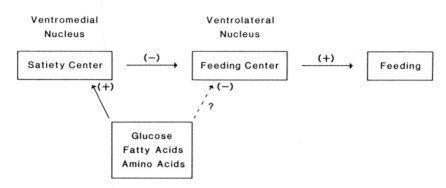

FIGURE 2–1.   Hypothalamic control of feeding.

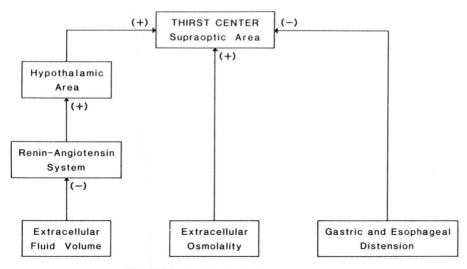

FIGURE 2–2.   Hypothalamic control of thirst.

this response. Hypovolemia results in an increased renin secretion, thereby producing an elevated circulating level of angiotensin II. The angiotensin II acts on specific areas of the hypothalamus which, in turn, activate the thirst center. Thus, hemorrhage leads to increased drinking despite an unchanged extracellular fluid osmolality.

Although the hypothalamic centers are the principal physiologic controllers of fluid intake, afferent nervous signals from the oropharynx and stomach also influence the thirst center. This fact is demonstrated by the relief of thirst immediately following fluid ingestion, even in patients with esophageal fistulae in whom the fluid does not reach the G.I. tract and therefore is not absorbed. Furthermore, simple distention of the stomach with a balloon affords transient relief of thirst. Perhaps these mechanisms serve to prevent excessive ingestion of fluid during the period of time required for absorbed fluid to correct the disturbances of extracellular osmolality and volume.

SALIVARY GLANDS

Saliva is important to the hygiene and comfort of the teeth and mouth and contributes to the normal digestion of food. Saliva is the product of a hetero-geneous group of exocrine glands which drain into the mouth. The three main pairs of salivary glands are the parotid, submandibular (submaxillary), and sublingual glands. In addition to these glands, there are numerous smaller glands located in the lips (labial glands), palate (palatine glands), tongue (lingual glands), and cheeks (buccal glands). The salivary glands are characterized by the nature of their secretions. The largest of the glands, the parotids, as well as the lingual glands, secrete a watery nonviscous solution (serous) containing primarily water and electrolytes. All of the other glands secrete a more viscid solution, the viscosity being due to the presence of mucins in the serous se-cretion. The glands producing this type of saliva are commonly referred to as mixed mucus and serous glands. The contributions of the parotid, submandib-ular, and sublingual glands to total output of saliva are estimated to be 20, 60, and 20 per cent, respectively.

The microscopic structure of the salivary glands is illustrated in Figure 2–3. The functional secretory unit of the salivary gland (sometimes referred to as the salivon) consists of the acinus, the intercalated duct, the striated duct, and the excretory (collecting) ducts. The acinus, the primary secretory unit, is a blind-end sac lined by large pyramidal cells. These cells are of either the serous or the mucous type. The serous cell is characterized by secretory gran-ules and a pronounced rough endoplasmic reticulum, features common to pro-tein-secreting cells. In contrast, the mucous cells contain histochemically de-monstrable mucous droplets and a sparse, rough endoplasmic reticulum. Lying between the secretory cells and their basement membrane are stellate-shaped myoepithelial cells which contain contractile elements. These cells are thought

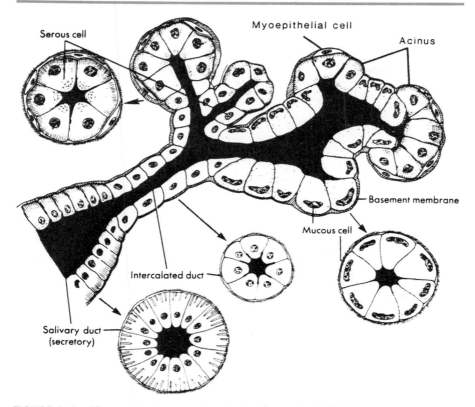

Serous cell

Myoepithelial cell

Acinus

Basement membrane

Mucous cell

Intercalated duct

Salivary duct
(secretory)

FIGURE 2–3. Microscopic structure of a mixed salivary gland. (Modified from Berne, R.M., and Levy, M.N.: Physiology. St. Louis, C.V. Mosby, 1983, p. 770.)

to compress the acinus and propel the primary secretions into the intercalated duct.

The intercalated ducts, so-called because they lie between the acinus and the striated duct, are lined by low cuboidal epithelium. They are also surrounded by myoepithelial cells which, upon contraction, further facilitate the movement of secreted fluid between the acinus and striated duct. Whether the acinar secretions are modified within the intercalated duct remains uncertain.

The striated ducts are lined by simple columnar epithelial cells. The striated appearance of the ducts is attributed to the characteristic infoldings of the basal cell membrane and the columns of mitochondria contained within these folds. The epithelial cells of the striated duct modify the ionic composition and osmolality of the acinar secretions. The larger excretory ducts are also lined

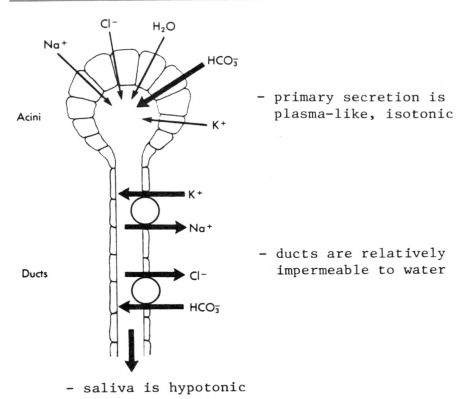

- primary secretion is plasma-like, isotonic

- ducts are relatively impermeable to water

- saliva is hypotonic

FIGURE 2–4. Water and electrolyte transport in the salivary unit. (Modified from Berne, R.M., and Levy, M.N.: Physiology. St. Louis, C.V. Mosby, 1983, p. 772.)

by columnar epithelium, and there is evidence that these structures may further modify the composition of saliva.

WATER AND ELECTROLYTE SECRETION

The acini are the primary sites of elaboration of saliva (Fig. 2–4). An isotonic or slightly hypertonic solution is produced by the acinar epithelium. This primary secretion is plasma-like in composition. It is probable that the secreted fluid is elaborated primarily by active electrolyte transport into the acinar lumen. However, a filtration component has also been invoked. Fluid collected by micropuncture from the intercalated duct is isotonic, implying that the primary secretion is either isotonic and therefore unmodified by the intercalated duct, or it is hypertonic, and osmotic equilibration occurs within the intercalated duct.

Salivary fluid at the level of the excretory ducts is hypotonic, indicating that some modifications of the primary secretion occur as it passes through the striated and excretory ducts. The striated and excretory duct epithelium actively absorbs sodium. The observation that the electrical potential difference (-70 mv, lumen negative) across ductal epithelium can be abolished by replacing sodium in the ductal fluid with choline or by sodium transport inhibitors such as ouabain lends support to the notion that the sodium is actively transported. The capacity of the ductal epithelium to transport sodium is demonstrated by observations that intercalated duct sodium concentration is 100 to 130 mEq per liter, while the sodium concentration in saliva obtained at the excretory duct opening is 10 to 30 mEq per liter. In contrast to sodium, potassium and bicarbonate are actively secreted by the ductal epithelium into the lumen. Chloride ions move out of the duct lumen either in exchange for bicarbonate or by passive diffusion along an electrochemical gradient (accompanying sodium) or both. The lateral intercellular channels of ductal epithelium are considered to be relatively impermeable to chloride ions; therefore, passive absorption of chloride lags behind the active absorption of sodium. Although electrolytes are both absorbed and secreted by the ductal epithelium, the net movement of ions is from lumen to blood. In spite of the osmotic gradient developed by the net outward movement of ions from the lumen, relatively little water is absorbed from the duct owing to the low permeability of the epithelial lining. The end result of these processes is that the primary secretion becomes hypotonic.

The degree of hypotonicity and the electrolyte composition of saliva are dependent upon the rate of salivary secretion (Fig. 2–5). At low secretion rates (0.5 ml/min), the movement of the primary secretion within the ducts is slow enough to allow the ductal transport processes to decrease the osmolality of the primary secretion by 70 per cent, i.e., to 88 mOsm per liter. This fluid contains approximately 10 mEq per liter of chloride and 26 mEq per liter of sodium, bicarbonate and potassium. As secretion rate is increased, the reduced time of exposure of the primary secretion to the ductal epithelium limits the amount of electrolytes which can be removed (sodium) or added (potassium). Thus, at higher secretion rates, the tonicity of the saliva approaches that of the primary secretion. For example, at a secretion rate of 4 ml/min (approximately 10 times the resting value), the osmolality of the saliva is approximately 212 mOsm per liter with the following ionic composition: sodium, 90 mEq per liter; bicarbonate, 58 mEq per liter; chloride, 46 mEq per liter; potassium, 18 mEq per liter. Although the dependence of ionic composition on secretion rate varies from one salivary gland to another, a common feature of all secretions is the relatively high content of potassium and bicarbonate at high secretion rates.

Substances which influence the secretory activity of salivary epithelium, such as hormones and neurotransmitters, do so by interacting with specific

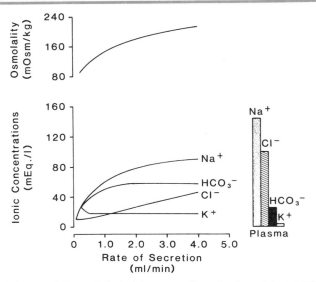

FIGURE 2–5.   The osmolality and electrolyte composition of salivary juice at different rates of secretion. Plasma levels of electrolytes are given for reference. (Modified from Thaysen, J.H., Thorn, N.A., and Schwartz, I.L.: Excretion of sodium, potassium, chloride and carbon dioxide in human parotid saliva. Am. J. Physiol., *178*:155, 1954.)

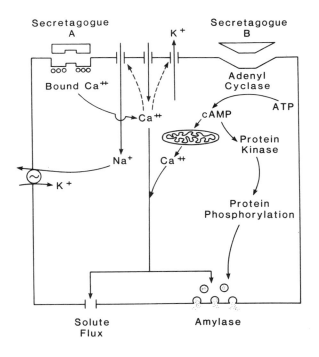

FIGURE 2–6. Stimulus-secretion coupling in the salivary gland.

membrane receptors. The cellular events which link receptor activation and secretion are termed "stimulus-secretion coupling" (Fig. 2–6). Interaction of a secretagogue with its receptor results in an increased permeability of the cell membrane to certain ions which, in turn, alter the resting membrane potential. In acinar cells, secretagogues increase membrane permeability to potassium, resulting in an efflux of cellular potassium. Consequently, the membrane potential changes from a resting value of -25 mv to -60 mv, i.e., hyperpolarization. This electrical response is in contrast to the events in ductal epithelium where secretagogues cause membrane depolarization, i.e., from a resting value of -70 mv to approximately -40 mv. Increased membrane permeability and subsequent intracellular accumulation of sodium ions may account for the depolarization. The intensity of the change in resting membrane potential of acinar and ductal epithelia is directly related to secretagogue concentration.

These alterations in membrane potential stimulate water and electrolyte secretion. The link between the electrical and secretory events is poorly understood but appears to involve changes in the intracellular concentration of both calcium and cyclic nucleotides (cyclic AMP, cyclic GMP). The role of calcium in stimulus-secretion coupling is demonstrated by the observation that salivary glands depleted of calcium lose their ability to secrete water and electrolytes, yet retain their ability to respond electrically to secretagogues.

Saliva contains proteins in concentrations ranging between 100 and 300 mg/dl. Salivary proteins can be divided into two classes, those specifically secreted by salivary epithelium (e.g., amylase and mucoproteins) and those which gain access to saliva via filtration (plasma proteins). A wide variety of proteins with diverse biologic functions fall under the category of secreted proteins. These include enzymes such as α-amylase (ptyalin), lingual lipase, and ribonuclease; antibacterial agents such as muramidase (lysozyme), immunoglobulins (chiefly IgA), and lactoferrin; and mucoproteins, which include mucins and the ABO blood group substances. There also exist in saliva a number of proteins whose biologic significance is not certain; these include "R-protein," which binds dietary vitamin B_{12}, and epidermal growth factor, which stimulates gastric mucosal growth.

Quantitatively, the most important of the salivary proteins are amylase and mucins. Amylase is almost entirely derived from the parotid glands, while the mucins are formed primarily in the sublingual and submandibular glands. Mucin is the primary determinant of salivary viscosity. The viscosity of whole saliva is 2.9 centipoises, yet the viscosities of the secretions of the sublingual, submandibular, and parotid glands are 13.4, 3.4, and 1.5, respectively.

Amylase is synthesized and stored in the serous (acinar) cells of the salivary gland (primarily parotids) in the form of zymogen granules (Fig. 2–6). These granules are located in the apical portion of the cell, and their contents are discharged by exocytosis into the lumen in response to certain secretagogues. Interaction of secretagogues with membrane receptors leads to increased intracellular cAMP and calcium concentrations. Cyclic AMP may modulate the cellular calcium changes because it appears to mobilize intracellular stores of calcium. An influx of extracellular calcium is required for sustained amylase release in response to secretagogues. An important step in exocytosis is phosphorylation of membrane proteins, an event which requires calcium and cAMP.

The steps involved in the release of mucin from mucous cells are poorly understood. Stored droplets of mucin in the apical portion of the cell are probably discharged by exocytosis, and it is likely that events similar to those in the serous cell link the stimulus to secretion. The stimulus for secretion also promotes the synthesis of the secreted product by the cell.

REGULATION OF SALIVARY SECRETION

Nervous Regulation

PARASYMPATHETICS

All salivary glands appear to receive parasympathetic nerve endings, which originate from the superior and inferior salivary nuclei and the seventh and ninth nerves. Fibers destined for the parotid gland are contained in the ninth cranial nerve and synapse in the otic ganglion, from which postganglionic fibers in the auriculotemporal nerve terminate on acinar and ductal elements of the gland. Preganglionic fibers for the submandibular and sublingual glands, the chorda tympani, course with the seventh cranial nerve and synapse in the submaxillary ganglion, from which ganglionic fibers innervate the gland and blood vessels. Both acetylcholine and vasoactive intestinal polypeptide are found in vesicles in the cholinergic nerve terminals.

The parasympathetic nervous system is recognized as the most important physiologic regulator of salivary secretion. Taste and tactile stimuli excite the salivatory nuclei which, in turn, increase the impulse frequency of the parasympathetic nerves supplying the gland. As shown in Figure 2–7, the rate of saliva formation is dramatically increased by stimulation of parasympathetic nerves over a range 1 to 10 pulses per second, with maximal secretion rates obtained at frequencies greater than 10 pulses per second. Under resting conditions, the impulse frequency is usually less than 1 pulse per second and it can increase to 4 to 8 pulses per second during feeding. Thus, as a result of parasympathetic activation associated with feeding, the rate of salivary secretion increases by 4 to 8 times. Noxious stimuli (such as a sore in the mouth) can produce parasympathetic nerve impulse frequencies exceeding 8 pulses per second, thereby resulting in maximal salivary secretion.

The importance of the parasympathetics in controlling salivation is further demonstrated by the observation that section of all parasympathetic nerves to the parotid gland abolishes the secretory response to citric acid placed in the mouth. Since acetylcholine is the neurotransmitter released at parasympathetic nerve endings, anticholinergic agents such as atropine effectively inhibit sali-

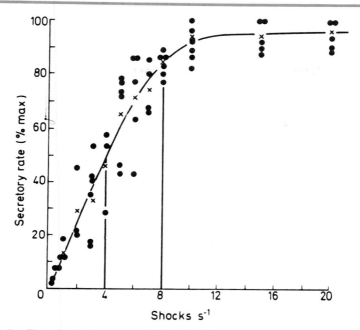

FIGURE 2–7. The effects of parasympathetic stimulation on salivary secretion. Vertical lines show the range of secretory rates when the glands were maximally activated by feeding. (From Emmelin, N., and Holmberg, J.: Impulse frequency in secretory nerves of salivary glands. J. Physiol. (Lond.), *191*:205, 1967.)

vary secretion. Furthermore, drugs (such as pilocarpine) that inhibit the activity of the enzyme cholinesterase, which degrades acetylcholine, enhance the rate of salivation.

SYMPATHETICS

The salivary glands are also innervated by sympathetic fibers. These fibers are derived from the first two thoracic segments via the superior cervical ganglion. The postganglionic fibers accompany the blood vessels into the glands, where they supply elements of the salivon (acini and ducts) and blood vessels. In contrast to the copious salivation elicited by parasympathetic stimulation, sympathetic stimulation produces a scant secretion. The maximal secretory rates produced by sympathetic stimulation are approximately one fifth the values observed with parasympathetic stimulation. The influence of sympathetic nerves on salivary secretion results primarily from activation of β-adrenergic receptors. Alpha-adrenergic receptors play a more important role in mediating the myoepithelial cell contraction associated with sympathetic stimulation.

TABLE 2–1.   Comparison of Sympathetic and Parasympathetic Influences on Salivary Secretion

Responses	Sympathetic	Parasympathetic
Saliva ouput	scant	copious
Temporal response	transient	sustained
Composition of secretions	protein rich, high K^+ and HCO_3^-	protein poor, lower K^+ and HCO_3^-
Response to denervation	decreased secretion	decreased secretion, glandular atrophy

Although both sympathetic and parasympathetic nerves are stimulants of salivary secretion, there are differences between the responses of the glands to the two neural influences (Table 2–1). Unlike parasympathetic stimulation, which produces a sustained copious flow of saliva, sympathetic stimulation produces a secretory response which tends to diminish or even cease despite continued stimulation. The composition of saliva is also dependent upon which division of the autonomic nervous system is stimulated. While the electrolyte composition of the acinar secretion is similar for the two neural influences, the saliva obtained from the main duct has a higher K^+ and HCO_3^- concentration, presumably indicating an effect of the sympathetics on the ductal epithelium. Another characteristic feature of sympathetically mediated secretion is a high protein concentration in the saliva. The myoepithelial cells are innervated by both divisions of the autonomic nervous system; however, the sympathetics appear to play a more important role in the contraction of acini and ducts, a process mediated by α-adrenergic receptors. Prolonged stimulation of either sympathetics or parasympathetics leads to salivary gland growth; however, parasympathetic denervation results in glandular atrophy, while sympathetic denervation does not. This fact presumably reflects a greater influence of the parasympathetics on basal salivary function.

Hormonal Regulation

In contrast to neural influences which affect all elements of the salivon, some hormones such as aldosterone and antidiuretic hormone exert their effects only on the ductal epithelium. Hormonal influences do not alter salivary secretion rate, yet they do modify the ionic composition of saliva. Aldosterone acts directly on the ducts to increase both sodium absorption and potassium secretion. Adrenocortical insufficiency is characterized by an increased salivary sodium concentration, while primary hyperaldosteronism and pregnancy (which is associated with high levels of mineralocorticoids) are characterized by a low sodium concentration in saliva. Antidiuretic hormone reduces the sodium concentration of saliva, presumably by enhancing sodium absorption in the ducts. The physiologic role of hormones in the regulation of salivary secretion appears, at present, to be far less important than that of neural influences.

Stimuli for Salivary Secretion

The most important stimuli for salivary secretion relate to events occurring before and during food ingestion. Even prior to ingestion, anticipation of food initiates salivation through signals from higher centers to the salivatory nuclei. This cephalic phase is reinforced by olfactory (smell) and visual stimuli. Salivation is not sustained unless food is eaten which activates proprioceptive (touch) and gustatory (taste) reflexes. Proprioceptive reflexes can be initiated by placing tasteless objects in the mouth, with smooth objects being more effective stimulants than rough ones. Of the gustatory stimuli, sour tasting or acidic material are the most potent.

Factors unrelated to food ingestion which decrease salivary secretion include sleep, anxiety, fear, mental effort, and dehydration. Nausea is associated with increased salivation, and the symptom of "water brash," which is the filling of the mouth with copious amounts of saliva, can occur in the presence of certain diseases of the upper G.I. tract, notably reflux esophagitis and duodenal ulcer.

FUNCTIONS OF SALIVA

Saliva serves several major functions, which can be broadly grouped into protective and digestive. The protective functions of saliva appear to be more important and can be attributed to the presence of various antibacterial agents, bicarbonate, and mucins. The human mouth is populated by a wide spectrum of pathogenic bacteria, which can cause dental caries and inflammation of the oral mucosa in the absence of saliva. The antibacterial action of saliva can be attributed to the presence of lactoferrin and muramidase (lysozyme). The iron-binding protein, lactoferrin, which is found in a number of exocrine secretions, including milk and pancreatic juice, exerts its action by depriving microorganisms of nutrient iron. Muramidase is a glycoprotein which hydrolyzes the muramic acid constituents of bacterial cell wall polysaccharides, thus destroying the microorganism. Immunoglobulins, which are capable of binding with antigenic components of the bacterial cell wall, are also present in saliva. However, their contribution to bacterial control in the mouth is unclear.

Bicarbonate, a major ionic constituent of saliva, plays an important role in the neutralization of acid in the mouth. The two major souces of acid in the mouth are ingested materials and the products of bacterial metabolism. Ingestion of acidic foods results in an increased secretion of saliva, which is rich in bicarbonate. This bicarbonate serves to partially neutralize the ingested acid. Acid released by bacteria plays an important role in the formation of dental caries (by dissolving enamel and dentine). In the absence of salivary bicarbonate, there is an increased incidence of dental caries. The buffering capacity of salivary bicarbonate is also important in the neutralization of gastric acid which is refluxed into the lower esophagus. Saliva also affords protection of oral structures between meals by providing a continual cleansing action in the mouth and by moistening the oral mucosa.

The contributions of saliva to digestion can be divided into lubricating properties and hydrolytic activities. The presence of mucins in saliva facilitates mastication and deglutition by diminishing the frictional interaction between the food bolus and the oral and esophageal mucosa. These functions are demonstrated by the observation that patients with inadequate salivary flows have difficulty in swallowing dry foods, even when they are taken with large amounts of water.

Salivary amylase hydrolyzes α-1,4 glycosidic bonds of polysaccharides such as starch. This enzyme cannot hydrolyze the β-linkages of cellulose. In the overall digestion of carbohydrates in man, salivary amylase plays only a minor role, owing to the limited time that the enzyme has to act under conditions close to its optimal pH (approximately 7.0). Although salivary bicarbonate helps in achieving the optimal pH, rapid entry of food into the acid environment of the stomach inactivates the enzyme. However, when food is chewed for an extended period of time, up to 75 per cent of the starch can be digested to the disaccharide stage by amylase in the mouth.

Another hydrolytic enzyme found in human oral secretions is lingual lipase. This enzyme can act at relatively low pH, and, therefore, it can continue its digestive activity in the stomach. Lingual lipase hydrolyzes triglycerides to fatty acids and mono- and diglycerides from the molecule. This enzyme initiates fat digestion but accounts for a minor proportion of overall fat digestion.

There are several other important functions of saliva. These include facilitation of speech, oral comfort, and taste, and modification of the temperature of ingested food. The moistening and lubricative properties of saliva are essential for oral comfort and clear speech. Inasmuch as gustatory function is enhanced by solubilization of foodstuffs, saliva facilitates taste sensation. The free flow of saliva dilutes and lowers the temperature of the ingested hot fluid, thereby preventing scalding.

SALIVARY BLOOD FLOW

The maximally stimulated salivary gland of the dog can secrete its own weight in saliva every two minutes (in man this requires 10 minutes). These high secretory rates create the need for high blood flows which provide the oxygen, nutrients, electrolytes, and water required for salivation. Blood flow to the salivary gland in man is provided by arterial vessels originating from the external carotid arteries. Blood vessels enter at the hilus of the glands and ramify within the parenchyma in accordance with the lobular structure, forming capillary plexuses around the acini and ducts. The plexuses of fenestrated capillaries surrounding the ducts are much denser than those surrounding the acini. Veins draining the salivary capillaries course with the arteries and exit the tissue at the hilus to finally drain into the external jugular vein. The classical view of the vascular arrangement within the salivary glands is that of a series-coupled portal network in which blood flows countercurrent to salivary flow. In this model, arterial inflow first supplies the ductular capillary network, which in turn drains via venules into the acinar capillary network, forming a portal system whose flow is countercurrent to salivary flow (Fig. 2–8). Such an arrangement would allow events occurring at the ducts to influence the function of the acini.

Resting blood flow in the salivary glands is comparable to that of other gastrointestinal organs (i.e., about 50 ml per min per 100 g) when expressed per unit mass of tissue. Blood flow to the salivary gland can increase tenfold in response to enhanced functional activity (secretion). This intense hyperemia compares with the 30 to 130 per cent increase in intestinal blood flow observed following a meal. The functional hyperemia in the salivary gland is associated with an increase in the number of perfused capillaries.

The possible mechanisms involved in the functional vasodilation of the salivary gland are illustrated in Figure 2–9. Although acetylcholine is clearly responsible for the secretory response to parasympathetic stimulation, the observation that atropine (anticholinergic agent) blocks the secretory response (but not the vasodilation produced by parasympathetic stimulation) indicates that it is not the mediator of the functional hyperemia. The most widely accepted mediator is bradykinin, a potent vasodilator that is derived from the proteolytic action of glandular kallikrein on plasma kininogen. The fact that atropine does not block the vasodilation induced by parasympathetic stimulation suggests that another neurotransmitter (e.g., VIP) is involved in the release of kallikrein. Vasoactive intestinal polypeptide and other noncholinergic neurotransmitters (e.g., substance P) may act directly on the vasculature to cause vasodilation. Metabolite accumulation has also been invoked to explain the vasodilation associated with enhanced salivary secretion. Such vasodilators might include adenosine, potassium ions, osmolality, and lactic acid.

The increased blood flow and perfused capillary density (capillary recruitment) associated with enhanced salivary secretion are essential for the maintenance of high rates of salivation. Arteriolar dilation leads to a rise in capillary hydrostatic pressure, which, coupled to the increased surface area for fluid exchange provided by capillary recruitment, allows for a greatly enhanced rate of capillary filtration. Thus, the fluid necessary for salivary secretion is provided by the circulation. The importance of the circulation in salivary secretion is demonstrated by the fact that, at high rates of secretion, the salivary venous hematocrit can increase from a value of 45 to 55 per cent owing to extraction of fluid from the blood. Furthermore, reductions in blood flow during maximal salivary stimulation lead to a reduction of secretion rate.

MASTICATION

Although chewing is not essential for the assimilation and digestion of foodstuffs, it does greatly facilitate these processes. Chewing is the process of

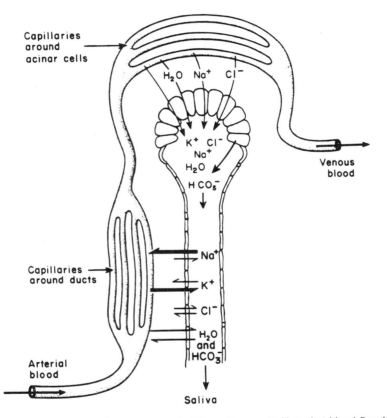

FIGURE 2–8. Microvascular arrangement of the salivary unit. Note that blood flow is countercurrent to salivary flow. Note also that the ductular capillary network drains into venules prior to perfusing the acinus (portal system). (Modified from Davenport, H.W.: Physiology of the Digestive Tract. Chicago, Year Book Medical Publishers, 1977, p. 93.)

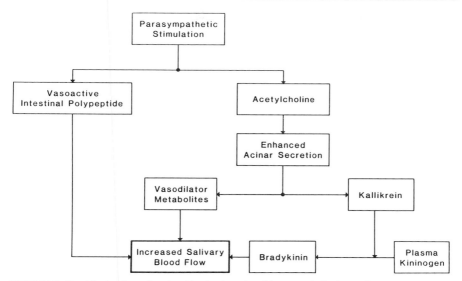

FIGURE 2–9. Mechanisms involved in the functional hyperemia in the salivary gland.

tearing, grinding, and cutting of solid food. It is accomplished by rhythmic muscular contractions which move the jaws to facilitate the frictional interaction between the food bolus and teeth. The tongue also takes part in this coordinated activity, moving the food along the surfaces of the teeth. The incisors provide a cutting and tearing action, while the molars grind food. The molars are capable of developing four times more pressure on food particles than are the incisors.

Chewing can be considered both a voluntary and an involuntary (reflex) activity. Stimulation of centers in the hindbrain can elicit and maintain chewing. Fibers from these centers run along the fifth nerve to supply the muscles involved in mastication. The two groups of muscles involved in chewing can be divided into those that open the mouth and those that close it. The masseter, medial pterygoid, and temporal muscles are involved in closing the mouth, while the lateral pterygoid and digastric muscles open the mouth. When a meal is ingested, the mouth, which is tonically closed, opens voluntarily. When the mouth is closed over a bolus of food, the pressure of food against the tongue, teeth, gums, and hard palate stimulates receptors which initiate the chewing reflex. The first event in the chewing cycle is relaxation of the jaw-closing muscles and contraction of jaw-opening muscles. This reduces the pressure exerted on the receptors and results in rebound relaxation of jaw-opening muscles and contraction of jaw-closing muscles. Muscle spindles in both groups of muscles act to coordinate the chewing process and to adjust tension development in jaw-closing muscles according to the consistency (hard vs. soft) of the food. In man, the duration of the chewing cycle is approximately one second.

Mastication serves several important functions related to food ingestion. Chewing not only stimulates salivary flow but also enhances the lubrication of food by mixing it with saliva. The carbohydrate component of many plant materials is encased in an indigestible fibrous (e.g., cellulose) coat. Chewing mechanically disrupts this coat, thus making the nutrient content available for digestion and absorption. Reduction of particle size of digestible foods by chewing facilitates the action of salivary and gastric enzymes by increasing the surface area available to these enzymes. Chewing and lubrication also protect the oral and esophageal mucosa from physical injury (abrasion) by hard and rough food particles.

DEGLUTITION

Swallowing (deglutition) usually begins as a voluntary act, but once initiated it proceeds through a reflex involving the coordinated action of the oral and pharyngeal musculatures (Fig. 2–10). The first step in this process (the voluntary stage) involves the separation of a portion of the food bolus in the mouth by lifting it with the tongue against the hard palate. The pressure exerted by the tongue then propels the bolus backwards toward the pharynx. When the bolus exerts pressure on sensory receptors near the opening of the pharynx, impulses are transmitted to the swallowing center in the medulla via various nerves (trigeminal, glossopharyngeal, and vagal). Stimulation of the swallowing center results in the coordinated contraction of a series of small pharyngeal muscles, resulting in a peristaltic wave which propels the bolus toward the upper esophagus. This motor activity involves various cranial nerves (fifth, seventh, ninth, tenth, and twelfth).

The passage of food through the pharynx (pharyngeal phase) involves the following sequence of events: the soft palate rises and the palatopharyngeal folds move inward, preventing nasopharyngeal reflux and creating a channel for the passage of the food bolus, respectively. Then the vocal chords are pulled together, and the epiglottis closes like a lid over the chords. At this point, respiration is inhibited and food is prevented from entering the trachea. The entire larynx is then pulled upward and forward, thus stretching the entrance to the esophagus. The pharyngeal phase ends with the opening of the pharyngeal-esophageal sphincter, thus allowing the food to enter the esophagus via pharyngeal peristalsis.

To summarize the mechanics of the pharyngeal stage of swallowing: the trachea is closed, the esophagus is opened, and a fast peristaltic wave originating in the pharynx then forces the bolus of food into the upper esophagus, the entire process occurring in 1 to 2 seconds.

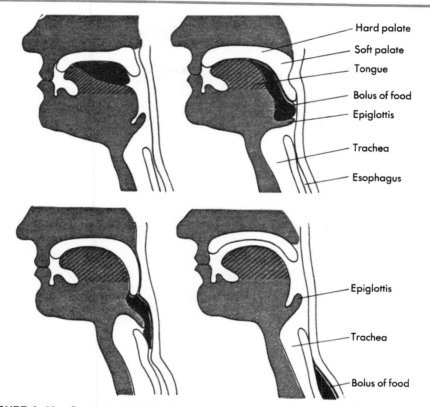

Hard palate

Soft palate

Tongue

Bolus of food

Epiglottis

Trachea

Esophagus

Epiglottis

Trachea

Bolus of food

FIGURE 2–10. Sequence of events involved in swallowing. (From Berne, R.M., and Levy, M.N.: Physiology. St. Louis, C.V. Mosby, 1983, p. 754.)

PAIN IN THE MOUTH AND OROPHARYNX

Unlike pain arising from the rest of the gastrointestinal tract, which involves autonomic nerves, pain from the mouth and oropharynx is conveyed by somatic nerves. The somatic nerves account for the fact that oral pain is not referred, but is localized to the affected area. The most common causes of pain in this region are dental and associated gingival diseases, ulcers of the oral mucosa, tonsillitis, and pharyngitis.

CLINICAL CORRELATIONS

Salivary Glands

The salivary glands can be affected by a number of pathologic processes, including inflammations and tumors. The most common inflammation is *mumps*, a viral infection which affects several tissues but has a predilection for the parotid gland. The inflammatory process, which produces vascular congestion and edema of the gland, results in marked swelling and pain. An old-fashioned home diagnostic test for the disease in its early stages is to give the child some lemon juice on his tongue. This provokes marked exacerbation of the parotid pain, presumably owing to an acute increase in congestion of the gland as reflex secretion, together with hyperemia, is provoked. Acid solutions such as lemon juice are particularly potent stimuli for salivary gland secretion.

The word "xerostomia" describes a chronic dry mouth. Several different diseases of the salivary glands can suppress salivary flow. One of these, *Sjögren's syndrome*, a condition related to rheumatoid arthritis, leads to failure of both lacrimation and salivation with dry eyes (xerophthalmia) and a dry mouth. Patients with xerostomia are prone to ulceration of the oral mucosa and severe dental caries. They also have great difficulty with chewing and swallowing; dry foods, such as crackers, are almost impossible to eat. These observations underscore the important role of saliva in lubrication of food for chewing and swallowing and its contribution to the integrity of oral structures by combating infection.

Deglutition

Given the complex and highly coordinated nature of the events involved in deglutition, it is not surprising that difficulty in swallowing (dysphagia) is a common consequence of diseases of the medulla oblongata; this area of the brain contains the swallowing center that regulates the activity of the cranial nerves such as the vagus. Diseases such as *bulbar poliomyelitis* and *progressive bulbar palsy*, a form of motor neuron disease, are frequently characterized by dysphagia. In some forms of bulbar polio it appears that the palatal muscles can function normally, and the dysphagia is attributed mainly to a fault in the coordinating mechanism, i.e., the swallowing center. In other cases, one can identify a disorder of a specific cranial nerve. Early in the swallowing sequence the nasopharynx is closed in order to prevent regurgitation of the food bolus into the nasal passages. This is achieved by the action of *levator veli palatini*, a muscle innervated by the vagus nerve. This muscle lifts the soft palate upward and backward, closing off the nasal passages. Most of the other small pharyngeal muscles involved in swallowing are also innervated by the vagus. Damage to the motor nucleus or fibers of one or both vagi will cause dysphagia, particularly for liquid foods. A prominent and very distressing feature of this dysfunction, particularly when both vagus nerves are involved, is nasal regurgitation of liquids. Difficulty in swallowing liquid food in such patients is a common cause of death as a result of choking and aspiration.

REFERENCES

Berne, R.M., and Levy, M.N.: Physiology. St. Louis, C.V. Mosby Co., 1983.
Davenport, H.W.: Physiology of the Digestive Tract. Chicago, Year Book Medical Publishers, 1977.
Schneyer, L.H., and Emmelin, N.: Salivary secretion. *In* Jacobson, E.D., and Shanbour, L.L. (eds.): International Review of Physiology: Gastrointestinal Physiology, I. Baltimore, University Park Press, 1974, pp. 184–226.
Young, J.A.: Salivary secretion of inorganic electrolytes. *In* Crane, R.K. (ed.): International Review of Physiology: Gastrointestinal Physiology, III. Baltimore, University Park Press, 1979, pp. 1–59.

The essential function of the esophagus is to transfer solids and liquids from the pharynx to the stomach. Although its main activity is related to eating and drinking, the esophagus occasionally functions to transfer gas (eructation) and gastric contents (vomiting) from stomach to mouth. The esophagus has no storage function and is normally empty and collapsed when not transferring material to the stomach. The esophagus does not have any digestive or absorptive abilities, and its only secretion is mucus, which serves to lubricate the food bolus as it passes to the stomach.

3

THE ESOPHAGUS

ANATOMIC CONSIDERATIONS

The esophagus is a hollow tube extending from the pharynx to the stomach. It is approximately 25 to 35 cm long in the adult human. At rest, it is empty and collapsed, its transverse diameter being approximately 3 cm and its anteroposterior diameter 2 cm. It is maintained empty by virtue of its two sphincters, the upper esophageal sphincter (UES) and the lower esophageal sphincter (LES). Both sphincters are defined operationally; i.e., they represent zones of high intraluminal pressure. The UES extends for about 3 cm at the junction of the pharynx and esophagus and appears to correspond to the cricopharyngeal muscle and the inferior pharyngeal constrictor. As the esophagus passes through the thorax, it lies in the posterior mediastinum, running in close apposition to the trachea and left main stem bronchus. The upper one third of the esophagus is surrounded by striated muscle, while the lower two thirds is composed of smooth muscle. There is a transition zone where both muscle types are found. There is no anatomic equivalent of the lower esophageal sphincter. Like the

53

UES, the lower sphincter is recognized as a zone of high pressure extending over a few centimeters close to the level of the diaphragmatic hiatus.

There is a sharp demarcation between squamous esophageal epithelium and glandular gastric mucosal epithelium, the squamocolumnar junction. In the collapsed esophagus, one can recognize this junction at endoscopy as a serrated line of demarcation which straightens out as the esophagus is distended. The esophageal mucosa appears as a pink featureless membrane with no obvious blood vessels. The mucosa consists of stratified squamous cells which account for up to 10 per cent of the total thickness of the layer. Extensions of the lamina propria into the epithelium are also seen. Some mucous glands are found in the lamina propria, particularly at the upper and lower ends of the esophagus; the ducts of these glands extend up through the squamous epithelium to the esophageal lumen. Under the lamina propria is the very thin muscularis mucosa which separates the mucosa from the submucosa, a zone of connective tissue. An inner circular and an outer longitudinal muscle layer lie beyond the submucosa. Auerbach's (myenteric) nerve plexus lies between these two muscle layers. Since the submucosa is very loose, the mucosa of the esophagus is free to move to some extent in relation to the esophageal muscle. Unlike other areas of the gastrointestinal tract, which have a peritoneal covering, there is no serosal coat on the muscle layer. This makes esophageal surgery somewhat difficult; the peritoneum is very useful in helping to secure anastomoses in the stomach and intestine.

It is worthwhile considering the detailed anatomic arrangement of structures in the distal esophagus, in view of the frequency of clinical disorders affecting this region. The normal relations of the cardioesophageal junction are shown diagrammatically in Figure 3–1. At the upper end of the LES zone of high pressure, there is an occasional slight thickening of the circular muscle, which is called the inferior esophageal sphincter. Lying between this sphincter and the squamocolumnar junction is the vestibule, often termed the ampulla when demonstrated radiologically. A portion of the LES lies below the diaphragm, and this part is exposed to intra-abdominal pressure, while the supradiaphragmatic portion is exposed to intrathoracic pressures.

As with much of the rest of the gastrointestinal tract, the most important nerve supplying the esophagus is the vagus, although the spinal accessory nerve supplies the high cervical esophagus. Where vagal afferents supply striated muscle in the upper esophagus, the nerves do not belong to the autonomic nervous system but terminate at motor end-plates. In the distal esophagus, parasympathetic vagal fibers synapse in Auerbach's plexus, from which short postganglionic nerve fibers arise to supply the two muscle layers. Sympathetic nerves arising from the cervical and thoracic chain ganglia also supply the esophagus. Little is known about esophageal afferents. Myelinated fibers which chiefly travel with the sympathetic nerves carry sensory information from the lower esophagus, while sensation from the upper esophagus is carried by parasympathetic fibers.

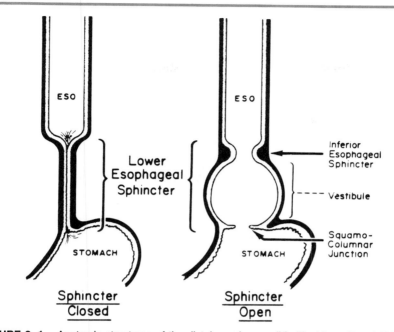

FIGURE 3–1. Anatomic structures of the distal esophagus. (Modified from Goyal, R.K., and Cobb, B.W. *In* Johnson, L.R. (ed.): Physiology of the Gastrointestinal Tract. New York, Raven Press, 1981, p. 362.)

ESOPHAGEAL FUNCTION

The Interdigestive Period

Two methods that are routinely used for studying esophageal activity are (1) cineradiography, which follows the transit of a swallowed bolus of barium through the esophagus, and (2) intraluminal pressure recording by manometry. The latter method utilizes small pressure transducers at the tip of a catheter or a perfused catheter system. The perfused catheters are usually about 2 mm in diameter and a combined recording device is made from four or five such catheters lashed together with their orifices at a set distance apart, e.g., 5 cm. The perfused catheter system allows for measurement of sequential pressures over a long segment of the esophagus, and it is used to estimate the speed of propagation of a peristaltic wave.

At rest, manometric measurement of pressures in the upper esophageal sphincter zone (2 to 4 cm) gives values in man of 40 to 100 mm Hg. Electrical recordings from the UES in the opossum, an animal whose esophagus resembles that of man, shows continuous electrical spike activity at rest. The basal electrical activity is responsible for the sustained muscle contraction and high intraluminal pressures at the UES. Vagal stimulation causes contraction of UES

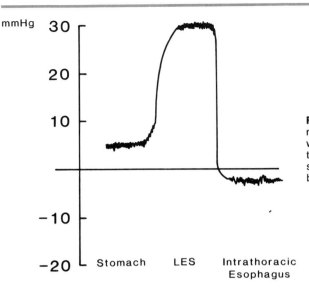

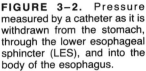

FIGURE 3–2. Pressure measured by a catheter as it is withdrawn from the stomach, through the lower esophageal sphincter (LES), and into the body of the esophagus.

muscles while vagal section abolishes their activity, indicating that parasympathetic nerve activity contributes significantly to basal tone of the UES.

In the body of the esophagus, the intraluminal pressure is related to respiration, being -5 to -15 mm Hg during inspiration and -2 to $+5$ mm Hg during expiration. Since intraesophageal pressure correlates well with intrapleural pressure, pulmonary physiologists use esophageal pressure as an indirect measure of intrapleural pressure. The position and pressures of the lower esophageal sphincter region are also affected by respiration. If one gradually withdraws a manometric catheter from the stomach (Fig. 3–2), the pressure rises from normal intragastric levels of 4 to 10 mm Hg to approximately 15 to 35 mm Hg over a distance of about 4 cm, then falls to the negative values of the body of the esophagus. Pressures in the upper and lower halves of the LES are affected differently by respiration. Inspiration causes an increase in pressure in the lower half and a fall in pressure in the upper half. The effect of respiration on the measured values of LES pressure is understandably complex. The LES moves axially with respiration. The vertical movements of the diaphragm alter, in a cyclical fashion, the external pressures exerted on the esophagus (positive intra-abdominal pressure and negative intrathoracic pressure).

There is continuous electrical spike activity in the LES under resting conditions, although a considerable amount of tone remains in the sphincter in the absence of this spike activity. It is probable that parasympathetic postganglionic cholinergic neurons contribute to LES tone, since muscarinic agents cause contraction in man and animals; on the other hand, atropine reduces it. The hormone gastrin was once believed to play a major role in maintaining the normal resting LES pressure, since exogenous doses cause contraction of the

TABLE 3–1.   Agents and Conditions Affecting Lower Esophageal Sphincter Pressure

Increase	Decrease
Protein meal	Chocolate
Coffee	Alcohol
Alkali	Peppermint
Gastrin	Smoking
Motilin	Gastric acidification
Prostaglandins	Secretin
Metoclopramide	Glucagon
Methacholine	Cholecystokinin
Bethanechol	Isoproterenol
Betazole	Atropine

sphincter. Careful evaluation of the form and concentration of circulating gastrin suggests that this is not the case. A wide variety of agents (Table 3–1) are known to affect LES pressure. Carminatives, agents which promote eructation and belching, were formerly used to relieve flatulence. Preparations such as mixtures of alcohol with ether (Hoffmann's drops) or with oil of peppermint reduce LES pressure and thus facilitate the escape of gas from the stomach. It can be seen from Table 3–1 that our after-dinner habits of smoking, drinking alcohol, and eating chocolate will all lower LES pressure and promote belching.

The Ingestive Period

Swallowing is a highly complex set of events controlled by a "swallowing center" in the medulla. Swallowing begins at 12 weeks intrauterine life. Normal adults swallow about 600 times per day, 350 times while awake, and 50 times during sleep. The remaining 200 times accompany eating and drinking. It is self-evident that respiration and swallowing should be closely coordinated. About 80 per cent of solid and liquid swallows occur in expiration. This coordination depends on the interplay between medullary centers controlling swallowing and respiratory activity.

With each swallow, the UES relaxes; its pressure may fall to subatmospheric levels, although not as low as esophageal values. The period of relaxation lasts 0.5 to 1.0 second and is followed by a period of enhanced pressure of approximately the same duration (Fig. 3–3). It can also be seen in this figure that there is a brief cessation of spike activity in the inferior pharyngeal constrictor and cricopharyngeal muscles associated with UES relaxation. This brief cessation is due to central inhibition rather than the activity of intrinsic inhibitory nerves, thus contrasting with the relaxation of the LES (see below).

In the body of the esophagus, the major motor event associated with swallowing is *primary peristalsis*, which is the continuation of oral and pharyngeal swallowing movements. A ring of contraction creating a wave of high pressure lasting 2 to 4 seconds travels at a speed of 3 to 5 cm per second, the greatest velocity being reached in the midesophagus (Fig. 3–4). The velocity of peristalsis with warm fluids is greater than with cold ones. The pressures

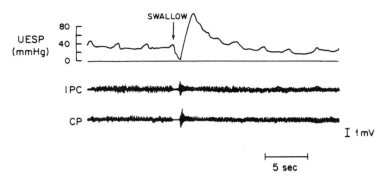

FIGURE 3–3. Sequential records of upper esophageal sphincter pressure (UESP) and myography (inferior pharyngeal constrictor (IPC) and cricopharyngeus (CP)). Note the cessation of spike activity in the muscles during swallowing and the increase in discharge afterwards, accompanied by a brief rise in UESP. (Modified from Goyal, R.K., and Cobb, B.W. *In* Johnson, L.R. (ed.): Physiology of the Gastrointestinal Tract. New York, Raven Press, 1981, p. 370.)

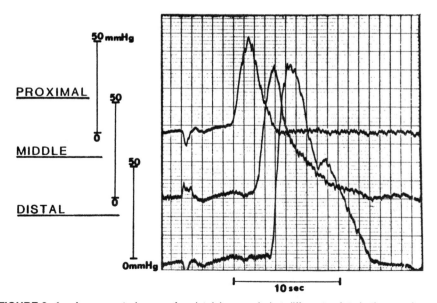

FIGURE 3–4. A propagated wave of peristalsis recorded at different points in the esophagus. Note the single high pressure wave traveling distally. (From Pope, C.E. *In* Sleisenger, M.H., and Fordtran, J.S. (eds.): Gastrointestinal Disease: Pathophysiology, Diagnosis, Management, 3rd ed. Philadelphia, W.B. Saunders, 1983, p. 421.)

FIGURE 3–5. Pressures in a normal human esophagus during a swallow. The start of the swallow is the deflection on the myograph (jaw muscles) tracing. Note the relaxation of the LES beginning almost at the start of swallowing, and the positive pressure change following relaxation. Note also the propagation of the peristaltic wave. (From Davenport, H.W.: Physiology of the Digestive Tract. Chicago, Year Book Medical Publishers, 1977, p. 14.)

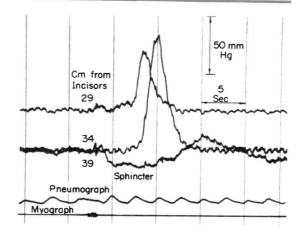

generated lie roughly between 35 and 70 mm Hg. The higher values are found in the upper and lower esophagus, while the lowest values are recorded in the region where the striated muscle blends with smooth muscle. The peristaltic wave does not pass through the LES; it reaches it approximately 6 seconds after swallowing begins. If a bolus of barium is swallowed, the peristaltic wave follows the tail of the bolus; i.e., it propels the bolus forward.

The LES relaxes in conjunction with swallowing (Fig. 3–5). The relaxation may begin at the start of deglutition but generally does not occur until about 2 seconds after the initiation of swallowing. A low viscosity bolus swallowed in the upright position may reach the LES with the help of gravity before relaxation has begun, and a transient delay results before the bolus enters the stomach. Relaxation of the LES is a much longer event (5 to 10 seconds) than that of the UES. Like the UES, relaxation is accompanied by a cessation of the continuous spike activity which occurs at rest. After relaxation, the upper half of the LES develops an after-contraction of 5 to 10 seconds while the lower half returns directly to the resting pressure level, as clearly shown in Figure 3–6.

Relaxation of the LES is a neurally mediated (vagal) reflex. Unlike relaxation of the UES, LES relaxation is not due to central inhibition of ongoing activity in the central nervous system but to release of an inhibitory neurotransmitter at the neuromuscular junction by postganglionic neurons. The transmitter has not yet been identified. It is not a cholinergic or adrenergic mechanism and is probably not purinergic. Some evidence suggests that vasoactive intestinal polypeptide may be responsible.

Secondary peristalsis is the term applied to the peristaltic waves which are initiated in the esophagus by afferent impulses from the esophagus itself. Unlike primary peristalsis, secondary peristaltic waves are not the consequence of the oropharyngeal movements of swallowing. They create no appreciable sensation. They seem to be responsible for clearing the esophagus of retained food material or refluxed gastric content. Distention is a particularly effective

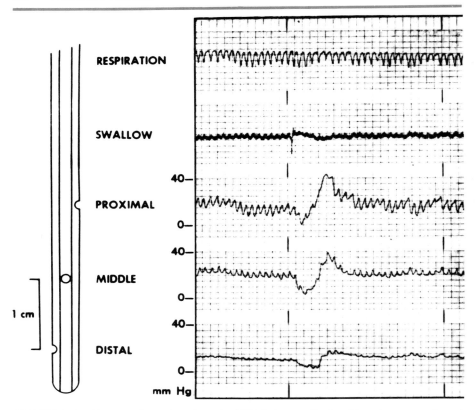

FIGURE 3–6. Manometric tracings from the LES during swallowing. The after-contraction of the upper two thirds of the sphincter is clearly shown. (From Pope, C.E. *In* Sleisenger, M.H., and Fordtran, J.S. (eds.): Gastrointestinal Disease: Pathophysiology, Diagnosis, Management, 3rd ed. Philadelphia, W.B. Saunders, 1983, p. 418.)

stimulus, since secondary peristalsis can be elicited by inflating a balloon in the body of the esophagus. The term tertiary contractions is chiefly used in a clinical setting. It usually denotes a series of simultaneous contractions in the body of the esophagus, often occurring spontaneously.

Under certain circumstances, the oropharyngeal movements of swallowing can be dissociated from peristaltic activity in the body of the esophagus. During drinking, there is a series of rapid swallows of up to 1 per second. During this period, peristalsis is inhibited ("deglutitive inhibition") by the sequence of closely spaced swallows. In addition, the LES remains relaxed during drinking, presumably as a result of inhibitory neuron discharge. The last swallowing movement during drinking, however, results in a peristaltic wave which empties the esophagus; then the LES resumes its resting pressure. For beer-swillers, the process of fluid transfer through the esophagus is much more efficient than drinking. In these individuals, the head and neck are extended, the larynx and pharynx descend, and both sphincters remain open. A constant column of fluid is maintained, and this pours into the stomach under gravity. Rapid to and fro movements of the tongue and soft palate transfer the beer from mouth to pharynx. As with drinking, a final peristaltic wave clears the esophagus.

GASTROESOPHAGEAL REFLUX—ANTIREFLUX MECHANISMS

Since the pressure in the body of the esophagus is subatmospheric while the pressure in the stomach is 5 to 10 mm Hg, some barrier in the gastroesophageal region must prevent reflux. Although mucosal folds at the cardioesophageal junction acting like valves and the acute angle of insertion of the esophagus into the stomach have been proposed as contributing to the antireflux effect, the function of the LES is of prime importance. Secondary peristalsis can be regarded as a second line of defense, clearing the esophagus of refluxed material.

The phenomenon of receptive relaxation of the stomach allows relatively large volumes of food and drink to be accommodated with small pressure increases; however, large-volume meals and swallowed air can increase the gastroesophageal pressure gradient substantially. As intragastric pressure rises, the resting LES pressure also rises, probably as a result of a neural reflex.

When intra-abdominal pressure increases, unlike intragastric pressure, the force is applied both to the stomach and to that segment of the LES which lies below the diaphragmatic hiatus. For example, in deep inspiration or during the Valsalva maneuver (forced expiration against a closed glottis) the pressure gradient between the stomach and the sphincter is unchanged, thus preventing reflux. The pinching action of the diaphragm on the esophagus may also assist at the point of maximal inspiration. A rise in intra-abdominal pressure also provokes a reflex rise in pressure throughout the entire LES; thus several mechanisms combat the tendency for reflux in the face of raised intra-abdominal pressure.

Esophageal reflux is common in late pregnancy. In this situation, intra-abdominal pressure is raised, and no subdiaphragmatic segment of the esophagus can be distinguished. The antireflux mechanism, therefore, depends only on the reflex rise in sphincter pressure initiated by the raised intra-abdominal pressure. Hormonal factors (notably progesterone), which affect smooth muscles of various organs during pregnancy, also reduce LES tone in late pregnancy, with consequent reflux. Secondary peristalsis, frequently observed in symptomatic reflux, disappears after childbirth.

In infants, antireflux mechanisms, i.e., LES function and secondary peristalsis, do not exist, explaining why infants regurgitate so readily. The diaphragm may play a relatively greater role in the prevention of gastroesophageal reflux in infants.

THE ESOPHAGEAL CIRCULATION

In terms of blood supply and lymph drainage, the esophagus can conveniently be divided into three parts. The blood supply of the upper esophagus comes from branches of the inferior thyroid artery, while vessels from the left gastric artery supply the lower esophagus. The middle esophagus is supplied by vessels from the thoracic aorta. Venous blood from the upper one third drains into the superior vena cava, from the middle third to the azygos system, while the lower one third drains into the portal vein via gastric veins. There are important potential anastomoses between the latter two systems which open up when portal venous pressure rises, thus draining the high pressure gastric venous blood to the lower pressure azygos system; such distended collateral veins are called esophageal varices. The reverse can also happen; when the superior vena cava is obstructed, collateral flow can occur through esophageal veins from the systemic to the portal circulation. The lymphatics of the upper esophagus drain to neck glands, those of the midesophagus to mediastinal nodes, and those of the lower esophagus to gastric lymph glands.

ESOPHAGEAL PAIN

Pain from the body of the esophagus is characteristically felt in the retrosternal region and, if severe enough, radiates to the back in the interscapular area. From the upper esophagus, pain radiates to the neck, while pain from the lower esophagus is experienced in the region of the xiphisternum.

An important cause of esophageal pain is the condition called diffuse esophageal spasm (DES). This dysfunction of motor activity, sometimes triggered by very hot or cold fluids, is characterized by periodic attacks of severe retrosternal pain due to strong uncoordinated contractions of the esophagus (sometimes called tertiary contractions). The patient may become pale and sweaty, and the pain may radiate to the neck, face, and arms, all characteristics of myocardial ischemia. The fact that DES and myocardial ischemia may coexist in an older patient, and that nitroglycerine may also relieve the pain of DES, can create a common diagnostic problem in view of the differences in management and prognosis of these two diseases. Esophageal manometry is a useful diagnostic tool in this situation.

Heartburn, a retrosternal burning sensation, is a common phenomenon attributed to esophageal reflux of gastric acid. It is particularly frequent in late pregnancy and is often experienced after large meals, particularly in the recumbent or bending position. In heartburn sufferers, the discomfort can be reproduced by perfusing the esophagus with 0.1 N HC1 (the Bernstein test), which is used to answer the question: are the patient's symptoms due to reflux esophagitis? It is not clear whether the sensation of heartburn is the result of stimulating specific acid-sensitive nerve endings or is a reflex muscle spasm in the esophagus.

CLINICAL CORRELATIONS

Two esophageal conditions which demonstrate the importance of normal peristaltic activity and a normally functioning LES are scleroderma and achalasia. Scleroderma belongs to that group of diseases which are called connective tissue disorders. It is an uncommon disease. An early manifestation of the condition is an induration of the skin which particularly affects the hands and face. The fingers become encased in tight, shiny, thickened skin which limits movements. Similarly, the facial skin becomes tight, restricting the opening of the mouth and obliterating the normal skin creases such as those of the forehead. A number of important internal organs can be affected, notably the heart and kidneys, resulting in the life-threatening complications of the disease. The gastrointestinal tract is also affected, particularly the esophagus and small intestine. Scleroderma of the esophagus results in a loss of peristaltic activity in the distal two thirds; thus there is no propagation of a peristaltic wave from the upper one third. The esophagus, therefore, behaves as a rigid tube. It would be reasonable to assume that the same excessive fibrous tissue deposition which occurs in the skin is responsible for the rigidity and lack of motility in the esophagus. Indeed, fibrosis is found, but the loss of peristalsis often precedes the development of fibrosis of the esophageal wall; thus some neuromuscular disorder seems to be responsible.

In patients with scleroderma, the lower esophageal sphincter becomes incompetent, and there is free reflux of acid gastric content into the lower esophagus, resulting in severe inflammatory changes in the mucosa (reflux esophagitis). Manometry demonstrates that there is reduced strength in the LES, sometimes to the extent that no high pressure zone can be demonstrated. Interestingly, the LES can respond normally to methacholine, a cholinergic agent, by contracting. Thus, there is a normal response to a direct muscle stimulant. However, there is an impaired response to edrophonium, an anticholinesterase; this suggests that there is a defect of the neurologic control of the sphincter, rather than of a muscle defect. On x-ray, the reflux of gastric content can be visualized with barium, and one may see air in the esophagus, which is normally collapsed and empty. It appears as if the stomach and esophagus behave as one continuous cavity. This can be confirmed by manometry. Normally, on inspiration, the diaphragm descends and intragastric pressure rises, while esophageal pressures fall as intrathoracic pressure falls. This pattern of pressure changes during respiration is lost in scleroderma.

Achalasia, once called cardiospasm, is a disorder of esophageal motility which affects both the LES and the lower two thirds of the body of the esophagus. Achalasia generally affects people between 20 and 40 years of age. The patient notices progressive difficulty in swallowing both solids and liquids. Pressure in the LES is usually markedly elevated, and the sphincter fails to relax adequately in response to swallowing. Organized peristaltic waves in the smooth muscle portion of the esophagus are absent. Thus, the fluid or food bolus is not propelled forward, and swallowed material is held up by the zone

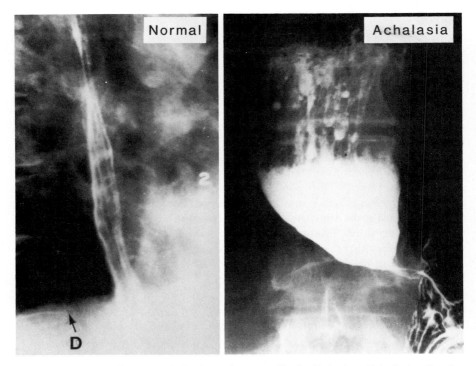

FIGURE 3–7. *Left,* The normal distal esophagus outlined with barium. D indicates the diaphragm. The faint parallel lines in the opacified esophagus represent normal longitudinal mucosal folds. *Right,* The distal esophagus in a 42-year-old man with achalasia. The esophagus is grossly dilated and filled with barium, fluid (saliva and esophageal secretions), and food particles. Note the smoothly tapered narrowing at the lower end of the esophagus.

of high pressure at the sphincter. Food only enters the stomach when the column of esophageal content is sufficiently high to overcome, by gravity, the resistance of the sphincter. The esophagus is often greatly dilated, and there is a constant risk that esophageal contents will be aspirated into the trachea. The esophageal mucosa usually shows inflammatory changes due to chronic stasis of food material.

On x-ray examination, swallowed barium, mixed with food particles and fluid, is seen being held up in the esophagus above a smoothly tapered constriction at the level of the LES (Fig. 3–7). Normally, a little swallowed air is seen in the fundus of the stomach on x-ray, but this is frequently absent in achalasia.

Manometry shows that the resting pressure of the LES is elevated and that it only partially relaxes (e.g., from 50 mm Hg to 35 mm Hg) in response to swallowing. Recordings from the body of the esophagus show no conducted peristaltic waves, but random low pressure activity is often seen. Both the body and the LES contract strongly with methacholine, and this has been regarded as a sign of "denervation hypersensitivity" and interpreted as evidence of a neurologic cause for this disorder. It is of interest that the LES is also hypersensitive to gastrin. There is histologic evidence of a neurologic problem, since there are reduced numbers of ganglion cells of Auerbach's plexus in the body of the esophagus and also in the region of the LES. Alterations in the motor (vagal) fibers supplying the esophagus have also been observed.

The treatment of this condition rests on mechanical disruption of the muscle fibers of the LES region using dilators or by a longitudinal surgical incision of the muscle of the distal esophagus.

REFERENCES

Davenport, H.W.: Physiology of the Digestive Tract. Chicago, Year Book Medical Publishers, 1977.

Goyal, R.K., and Cobb, B.W.: Motility of the pharynx, esophagus and esophageal sphincters. *In* Johnson, L.R. (ed.): Physiology of the Gastrointestinal Tract. New York, Raven Press, 1981, pp. 359–391.

Pope, C.E.: The esophagus: Physiology. *In* Sleisenger, M.H., and Fordtran, J.S. (eds.): Gastrointestinal Disease, 3rd ed. Philadelphia, W.B. Saunders, 1983, pp. 414–423.

While the esophagus serves simply as a conduit for food on its rapid passage from oropharynx to stomach, the principal roles of the stomach are to store food and process it in a preliminary fashion prior to its entry into the small intestine. By regulating the delivery of food to the duodenum, the stomach protects the small intestine from being suddenly overwhelmed by the arrival of large amounts of poorly prepared material. While in the stomach, food undergoes substantial chemical and physical modification. During the hours after a meal, the small intestine receives a flow of gastric chyme, a semifluid mixture of solutes, emulsion particles, and suspended material which are the products of digestive activity of gastric juice and mechanical action of the stomach. A patient with a total gastrectomy must substantially modify his eating habits to compensate for the loss of storage and digestive functions of the stomach. Although the stomach is not an important absorptive organ, some water and lipid-soluble substances can be absorbed at this level of the gastrointestinal tract. Ethanol is an important example of a lipid-soluble substance which is rapidly and extensively absorbed by the stomach.

4

THE STOMACH

STRUCTURE OF THE STOMACH

As illustrated in Figure 4–1, the human stomach can be divided into a number of regions, which are functionally distinct. At the esophagogastric junction, the lower esophageal sphincter creates a barrier to reflux of gastric contents to the esophagus and thus functionally separates the esophagus from the stomach. At the lower end of the stomach is the pyloric sphincter, which separates the stomach from the duodenum. The pyloric sphincter is a well-defined ring of smooth muscle which is involved in regulating the passage of chyme into the upper small intestine.

When opened, the mucosal surface of the stomach appears to be thrown up in longitudinal folds (rugae) which are most conspicuous in the body of the stomach. Like other parts of the alimentary tract, the stomach wall consists of well defined tissue layers—the mucosal, submucosal, and muscle layers. On the outer surface of the muscle lies the serosal (or peritoneal) layer. While submucosal and muscle layers are essentially similar to those of other layers of

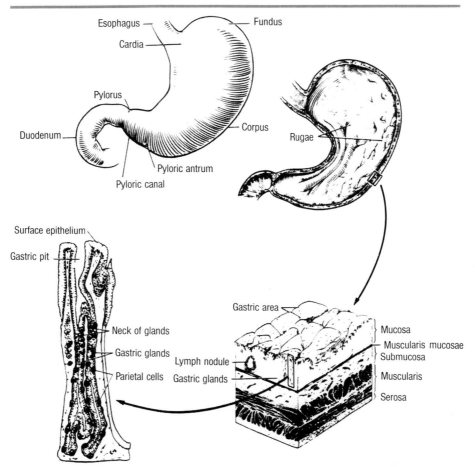

Esophagus

Fundus

Cardia

Pylorus

Duodenum

Corpus

Rugae

Pyloric antrum

Pyloric canal

Surface epithelium

Gastric pit

Gastric area

Mucosa

Neck of glands

Muscularis mucosae

Gastric glands

Submucosa

Lymph nodule

Parietal cells   Gastric glands

Muscularis

Serosa

FIGURE 4–1.   Macroscopic and microscopic anatomy of the stomach. (From Ito, S. *In* Johnson, L.R. (ed.): Physiology of the Gastrointestinal Tract. New York, Raven Press, 1981, p. 519.)

the gut, the gastric mucosa possesses a distinctive structure, which correlates with its various functions.

The epithelium of the gastric mucosa (Table 4–1) is chiefly concerned with secretory processes, i.e., the elaboration of gastric juice, a digestive mixture of hydrochloric acid, the enzyme pepsin, and mucus. The entire mucosal surface of the stomach is lined by a layer of simple columnar epithelium, the surface mucous cells, which secrete an alkaline solution of mucus. Mucus protects the gastric mucosa from chemical and physical injury. At the cardiac region there is an abrupt transition between surface mucous cells and the stratified squamous epithelium of the esophageal mucosa. The mucus-secreting cells also dip down from the surface to form the gastric pits, into which drain one or more gastric glands (Fig. 4–2). Mucous cells are also found in the neck of the glands. The

TABLE 4–1.   Epithelium of the Gastric Mucosa

Cell Type	Location	Secretion/Function
Mucous neck cell	primarily neck of gastric glands	produce mucus
G cell	glands in the pyloric antrum	produce gastrin
Parietal (oxyntic) cell	glands in the corpus	produce HCl and intrinsic factor (Vitamin B_{12}-binding protein)
Chief (peptic) cell	glands in the corpus	produce pepsinogen
Surface mucous cells	entire mucosa (except cardiac region)	produce mucus and alkaline secretion
Undifferentiated (stem) cells	gastric glands	replace surface mucous cells, and chief and parietal cells

mucous neck cells are larger than the surface mucous cells and produce a mucus which has distinctly different physicochemical characteristics from that produced by the surface mucous cells. Also located in the neck of the glands are the important undifferentiated (stem) cells which are constantly replacing the gastric epithelium, i.e., both the surface mucous cells and, at a slower rate, the chief and parietal cells. The potential for rapid division of these undifferentiated cells accounts for the ability of the gastric mucosa to repair itself after injury.

In that region of the stomach adjacent to the esophagus, a small area of mucosa contains the cardiac glands, consisting mainly of mucous cells and undifferentiated cells but no oxyntic or chief cells, which are characteristically found in the glands of the body of the stomach. The pyloric antral region, a much larger area than the cardiac region, contains glands which consist mainly of cells similar to mucous neck cells but, like the glands of the cardiac region, there are no oxyntic or chief cells. The pyloric glands, however, have numerous endocrine cells, the G cells, which produce the hormone gastrin.

The parietal or oxyntic cells have a conical shape and are found in the neck and deeper regions of the glands of the body of the stomach. These cells are the source of hydrochloric acid and the cobalamin-binding protein, intrinsic factor. Electron microscopy of these cells shows them to be full of smooth membranes termed tubular vesicles and numerous large mitochondria. It is estimated that the mitochondria occupy about one third of the volume of a parietal cell. Intracellular secretory canaliculi are prominent, and microvilli are found both in these canaliculi and at the luminal pole of the cell. The microvilli of the luminal membrane are much more numerous and elongated when the cells are actively secreting acid and greatly increase the surface area of the cell (Fig. 4–3).

The chief or peptic cell is found mostly in the deeper regions of the gland, and it is the source of pepsinogen. The morphology of the chief cell is very similar to that of the acinar cell of the pancreas (which also secretes enzymes),

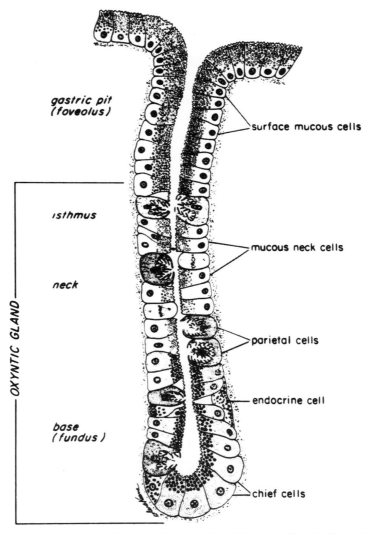

gastric pit
(foveolus)

surface mucous cells

isthmus

mucous neck cells

neck

parietal cells

endocrine cell

base
(fundus)

chief cells

OXYNTIC GLAND

FIGURE 4–2.   A gastric (oxyntic) gland. (From Ito, S. *In* Johnson, L.R. (ed.): Physiology of the Gastrointestinal Tract. New York, Raven Press, 1981, p. 520.)

being characterized by masses of rough endoplasmic reticulum and zymogen granules lying in the apical region of the cell. The chief cell discharges its products by exocytosis of the zymogen granules. The synthesis and intracellular transport of pepsinogen are very similar to the intracellular events in the pancreatic acinar cells.

Although a variety of hormones have been found in the gastric mucosa, the G, or gastrin cell, is the predominant endocrine cell found in the pyloric glands. This cell has a narrow apical membrane facing the gland lumen and is characterized by the presence of numerous secretion granules stored in the basal region of the cell.

Innervation of the Stomach

The extrinsic innervation of the stomach is via the parasympathetic division (vagus nerves) and the sympathetic, via the celiac plexus. In terms of function, i.e., secretion and motility, the parasympathetic supply is much more important. Nerve fibers end close to the various types of secretory epithelium and in the muscle layers. In addition, parasympathetic preganglionic and sympathetic postganglionic fibers synapse with the neurons of the myenteric and submucous plexuses, thereby influencing gastric functions.

GASTRIC JUICE

The stomach, both at rest and during activity, produces a unique secretion consisting of a solution of hydrochloric acid (HCl), the proteolytic enzyme pepsin, mucus, and electrolytes. This solution also contains intrinsic factor, which is necessary for vitamin B_{12} absorption. Lipolytic enzyme activity has also been found in gastric juice, but this activity is probably due to swallowed lipase derived from saliva. The electrolyte composition of gastric juice is variable, and this is best understood if one regards it as a two-component secretion, that is, an acid solution produced by the parietal cells and a nonacid juice produced by other gastric epithelial cells. The output of the acid component is highly variable, responding to various stimulating agents. If it is assumed that the rate of output of nonacid juice is constant and that the acid component is of constant composition, then it is possible to extrapolate from the composition of gastric juice secreted at different rates and derive the composition of the nonacid secretion, i.e., when there is no parietal cell contribution. The different rates of flow of gastric juice can be achieved by stimulating the stomach with secretagogues such as histamine. The calculated ionic composition of the nonacid component of the juice is somewhat similar to an ultrafiltrate of plasma (Table 4–2). However, it is distinctly alkaline owing to its high bicarbonate content, and it contains much more potassium than plasma. Furthermore, it contains mucus.

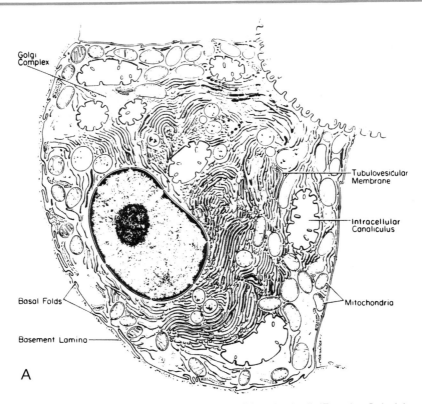

Golgi Complex

Tubulovesicular Membrane

Intracellular Canaliculus

Basal Folds

Basement Lamina

Mitochondria

A

FIGURE 4–3. The resting (*A*) and actively secreting (*B*) parietal cell. (From Ito, S. *In* Johnson, L.R. (ed.): Physiology of the Gastrointestinal Tract. New York, Raven Press, 1981, p. 531.)

Illustration continues on opposite page

The nonparietal alkaline secretion is believed to be derived from the surface mucous cells. These cells contain most of the gastric mucosal carbonic anhydrase, the enzyme which catalyzes the reaction of carbon dioxide and water to form carbonic acid, which dissociates, releasing bicarbonate (HCO_3^-) and hydrogen (H^+) ions. The production of an alkaline component of gastric juice is strongly depressed by acetazolamide, an inhibitor of carbonic anhydrase. The secretion of HCO_3^- by the mucous cells is an active process.

Mucus is the other important component of the nonacid secretion of the stomach. The main organic component of gastric mucus is a group of high molecular weight glycoproteins. Mucus is a gel which provides a flexible protective cover for the gastric mucosa. Direct observation of the mucosa shows that a continuous layer of mucus overlies the epithelial surface and that removal of a portion of it promptly stimulates the secretion of more mucus to repair the defect. The protective role of mucus for the mucosa is underlined by the

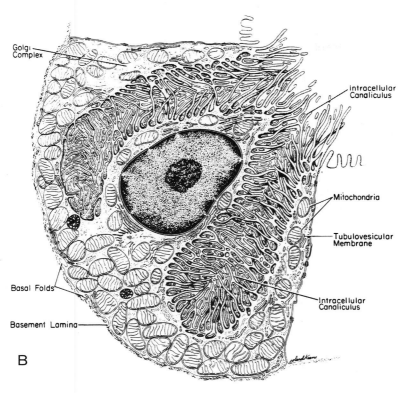

FIGURE 4–3. *Continued*

TABLE 4–2. Estimated Composition of Human Nonparietal Secretion

Electrolyte	Concentration
Na$^+$	150–160 mM
K$^+$	10–20 mM
Ca^{++}	3–4 mM
Cl$^-$	125 mM
HCO$_3^-$	45 mM
pH*	7.67

*pH estimated from HCO$_3^-$ concentration and an assumed Pco$_2$ = 40 mm Hg

fact that mechanical stimulation, such as rubbing or exposure to potentially injurious agents, provokes copious mucus secretion. It is possible that mucus and bicarbonate cooperate to protect the surface mucosal epithelium from injury by H^+. If the bicarbonate secreted by the surface epithelial cells were free in the lumen of the stomach, the H^+ secreted by the parietal cells would quickly overwhelm it. However, the HCO_3^- is somewhat immobilized in the surface mucus layer, creating an alkaline barrier to the diffusion of H^+ back to the epithelium. This creates a gradient of several pH units between the lumen ($\sim$ pH 2) and the surface of the mucosal cells ($\sim$ pH 6.5). There is considerable proteolytic activity in gastric juice due to pepsin; this enzyme degrades the superficial layers of gastric mucus but, at the same time, this degradation is offset by continuing secretion of fresh mucus by the underlying cells.

Pepsinogen is a proenzyme, or zymogenic form, of the powerful protease pepsin. The secretion and activation of pepsinogen is associated with the production of HCl by the stomach. Pepsinogen represents a family of proteins of approximately 42,000 molecular weight. Two groups, pepsinogens I and II, can be distinguished by electrophoresis. Both groups are found in the chief cells and, to some extent, in the mucous neck cells. Group II pepsinogens occur in the pyloric mucosa and in the Brunner's glands of the duodenum. Pepsinogen is rapidly converted to pepsin at pH 2; this activation involves splitting a peptide of approximately 7000 molecular weight from pepsinogen. At higher pHs, activation is progressively slower and, at pH 6, it is virtually abolished. Pepsin, once released, catalyzes its own conversion from pepsinogen, an example of a positive feedback mechanism. It cleaves proteins to peptides at aromatic amino acid links, reducing dietary proteins to a mixture of peptides. The optimum pH for pepsin activity lies between 1.8 and 3.5. Activity is lost at pH 7, and the enzyme is irreversibly destroyed in alkaline solutions. Stimulation of chief cells by food ingestion leads to degranulation of the cells, but continued synthesis of pepsinogen maintains the output of the enzyme. After a meal, it takes several hours for reaccumulation of the granules.

It is the HCl content of gastric juice which makes this digestive secretion so fascinating to physiologists and physicians. The contribution of HCl to digestive effort comes from acid digestion of foodstuffs, particularly in separating meat fibers by dissolving connective tissue and from its activation of pepsin. In a mixed meal, however, there are sufficient buffering agents such as proteins that intragastric pH rapidly rises from about 1 or 2 to 4 or 5 soon after food reaches the stomach. The growth of microorganisms, introduced into the stomach via fluids and foods, is limited by the secretion of hydrochloric acid. Overgrowth of various bacteria and other microorganisms is common in stomachs which do not secrete acid. In pathophysiologic terms, HCl and pepsin are potentially injurious to the mucosa of the esophagus, stomach, and duodenum and are the aggressive factors in the initiation of mucosal erosions and ulceration.

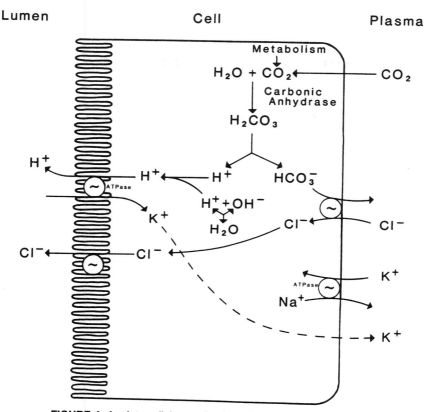

FIGURE 4–4. Intracellular mechanism of gastric acid secretion.

ELABORATION OF HYDROCHLORIC ACID BY THE PARIETAL CELLS

While the synthesis and secretion of pepsinogen and mucus by their cells of origin seem to follow patterns similar to other secretory cells, the production of HCl by the parietal cells is unique. The secretion from parietal cells is approximately 150 mN HCl and is isosmotic with plasma, but between plasma and the gastric lumen there is a huge gradient of H^+ (plasma: 0.00005 mN; parietal cell secretion: 150 mN). Transport against such a gradient involves an active process which requires ATP, generated by mitochondrial metabolism of glucose and fatty acids. Present evidence is consistent with the following sequence of events in the formation of HCl (Fig. 4–4): hydrogen ions for secretion are derived from the hydrolysis of water:

$$H_2O \rightarrow H^+ + OH^- \tag{1}$$

The essential transport mechanism is the H^+-K^+ exchange pump, which is located in the microvilli of the secretory canaliculi. Energy for the pump is provided by the enzyme, H^+,K^+-ATPase. Carbonic acid is generated within the parietal cell by the action of carbonic anhydrase on water and carbon dioxide:

$$H_2O + CO_2 \rightarrow H_2CO_3 \tag{2}$$

The H_2CO_3 dissociates into hydrogen and bicarbonate ions:

$$H_2CO_3 \rightarrow H^+ + HCO_3^- \tag{3}$$

The H^+ derived from carbonic acid reacts with hydroxide ions to form water, while HCO_3^- (Equation 3) leaves the basal pole of the cell in exchange for plasma Cl^-. The flow of HCO_3^- into gastric venous blood during parietal cell secretion raises the pH of the blood and is termed the "alkaline tide." The parietal cells actively transport Cl^- from the serosal side to the lumen. Thus, both ions of hydrochloric acid are actively transported to the juice. These ions take water with them by osmotic action (see Fig. 1–13 for discussion of the standing osmotic gradient theory). The transfer of Cl^- to the lumen is somewhat greater than that of H^+, the result being a potential difference across the gastric mucosa of 30 to 60 mv, the lumen being negative.

When the stomach is not secreting acid, Na^+ is actively transported from the lumen to the mucosa. This transport across the nonsecreting mucosa accounts for a potential difference of similar polarity to that which is found when hydrochloric acid *is* being secreted. This transport of Na^+ is inhibited during acid secretion. There is a close link between cellular potassium and acid secretion; while the stomach is secreting acid, the H^+,K^+-ATPase responsible for H^+ secretion maintains the concentration of intracellular K^+. When the stomach is at rest, intracellular potassium levels are controlled by Na^+,K^+-ATPases.

As described above, gastric juice is derived from two secretory processes: an acid secretion and a nonacid secretion. In the nonstimulated stomach, the nonacid component of gastric juice is the dominant secretion; therefore, the concentration of H^+ is low, and Na^+ is the predominant cation (Fig. 4–5). When the stomach is stimulated, the acid component becomes the dominant secretion. Therefore, the H^+ concentration rises, and there is a reciprocal fall in the Na^+ concentration (due to dilution of the nonacid secretion). At all rates of flow, K^+ and Cl^- concentrations tend to remain fairly constant.

STIMULI FOR GASTRIC SECRETION

Mucus secretion is chiefly stimulated by parasympathetic (vagal) activity. This vagal activity is also the main stimulus for pepsinogen secretion, although

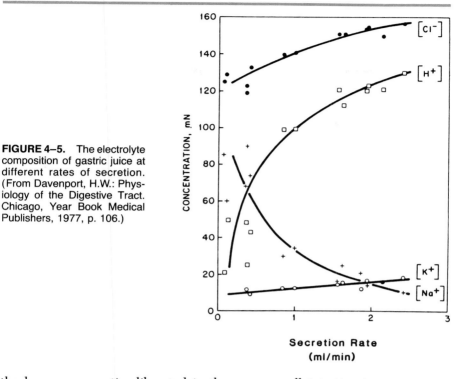

FIGURE 4–5. The electrolyte composition of gastric juice at different rates of secretion. (From Davenport, H.W.: Physiology of the Digestive Tract. Chicago, Year Book Medical Publishers, 1977, p. 106.)

the hormone secretin, liberated in the upper small intestine in response to duodenal acidification, also stimulates the chief cells. This action is greatly enhanced by acid in the gastric lumen. For the parietal cell, three principal stimuli have long been recognized: (1) acetylcholine released from parasympathetic nerve endings, (2) histamine derived from "mast-like" cells in the lamina propria of the gastric mucosa, and (3) gastrin. Receptors for each of these substances exist on the parietal cell membrane, and synergism occurs between these three agents. In general, agents which stimulate parietal cell secretion of acid also cause the release of intrinsic factor.

The parietal cell histamine receptor is termed an H_2-receptor, which distinguishes it from H_1-receptors found in other tissues such as bronchial smooth muscle. These two types of receptors recognize different parts of the histamine molecule. In the past, measurement of the acid-secreting ability of the stomach by stimulating the parietal cells with histamine required the simultaneous administration of an H_1-receptor blocking agent to prevent unwanted H_1 effects such as bronchoconstriction. The development in the past decade of potent H_2-receptor blocking agents such as cimetidine has revolutionized peptic ulcer therapy by controlled reduction of gastric acid secretion over a few weeks, allowing healing. The intracellular link between secretagogues such as histamine and acid secretion is the subject of much investigation. There is, at present, good evidence for one such link in this process, i.e., cyclic AMP.

SECRETORY CAPACITY OF THE STOMACH

In the unstimulated human stomach between meals, acid secretion is about 2 to 3 mEq per hour and seldom exceeds 5 mEq per hour. Stimulation with increasing doses of histamine or pentagastrin (a synthetic analogue of gastrin) results in progressively more acid secretion, until a maximum is reached. For pentagastrin, a subcutaneous dose of 6 μg/kg will maximally stimulate the human stomach, the peak flow occurring 15 to 45 minutes after injection. Peak acid output (as mEquivalents per hour) is obtained by multiplying by 4 the mEquivalents of HCl secreted during the 15-minute period of maximum secretion. The results from healthy subjects usually lie between 10 and 35 mEq per hour, values for men being higher than those for women. The maximum capacity of a stomach for HCl secretion correlates well with the total number of parietal cells. The hormone gastrin not only causes parietal cell secretion but, over a longer period of time, promotes growth of gastrointestinal tissues, notably the parietal cell mass (which is normally one billion cells). Exposure of the stomach to high sustained concentrations of gastrin leads to such growth, together with an increased peak acid output. This growth occurs in the rare pancreatic tumor, the gastrinoma, where high circulating levels of gastrin are found.

CONTROL OF GASTRIC SECRETION

The stomach secretes continuously (basal secretion), but superimposed on this are phases of stimulated secretion associated with feeding. The amount of hydrochloric acid secreted under basal (fasting) conditions, relative to the maximum secretory response to an exogenous stimulant like histamine or pentagastrin, varies with different species; in man, it is approximately 10 per cent of the maximum secretory rate. If the vagus nerves are cut (vagotomy), basal secretion is reduced. It is virtually abolished if the gastric antrum has also been removed. It is inferred, therefore, that basal secretion is maintained by a combination of background vagal activity and the secretion of gastrin. Basal secretion shows a circadian rhythm, being highest in the evening and low in the morning; what controls this rhythm is unknown.

The secretory response of the stomach to meals has traditionally (and conveniently) been divided into three phases: *cephalic* (stimuli involving the head), *gastric*, and *intestinal*. The *cephalic* phase is initiated by anticipation of eating, followed by the sight, smell, and taste of food, and is exclusively mediated by the vagus nerve, since, regardless of the stimulus, it is abolished by vagotomy. Sham feeding in the dog with an esophageal fistula will provoke this secretion, although no food enters the stomach. The magnitude of the secretory response is proportional to the period of sham feeding. There is no secretory response, however, when water is taken; thus the stimulus must be a nutrient. Vagally mediated gastrin release is considered to play a major role in the cephalic

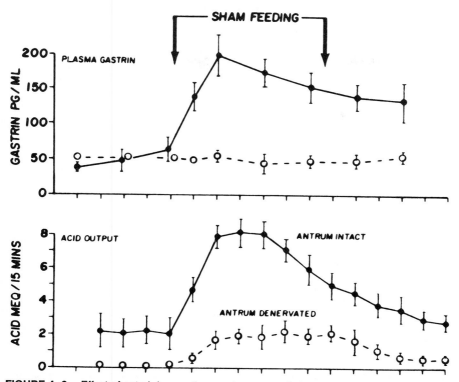

FIGURE 4–6.   Effect of antral denervation on plasma gastrin levels and gastric acid secretion in dogs with esophageal fistulae. Note that antral denervation, which eliminates vagally induced gastrin release, significantly attenuates the acid output in response to sham feeding (cephalic phase). (From Tepperman, B.L., Walsh, J.H., and Preshaw, R.M.: Effect of antral denervation on gastrin release by sham feeding and insulin hypoglycemia in dogs. Gastroenterology, *63*:973, 1972.)

phase (Fig. 4–6). Denervation of the antrum, which effectively eliminates vagally mediated gastrin secretion, significantly depresses acid output in the cephalic phase. In man, it is estimated that gastric acid secretion during the cephalic phase can increase to 40 per cent of the maximum secretory response of the stomach. Cephalic phase secretion can be simulated experimentally by reducing the glucose available to the brain, e.g., with insulin hypoglycemia or by giving the nonmetabolizable glucose analogue, 2-deoxy-D-glucose.

A conditioned reflex will also result in cephalic stimulation of gastric acid secretion. The classic experiments of Pavlov with dogs involved ringing a bell at the time of feeding. Eventually, the bell alone induced gastric secretion. The association can be "forgotten"; thus, to maintain the conditioned reflex, it is necessary to re-establish periodically the link between the bell and feeding.

The arrival of food in the stomach initiates the gastric phase of secretion by distention and by chemical actions of specific food components. Distention of the entire stomach enhances gastric secretion through neural mechanisms involving long vago-vagal reflexes, i.e., afferent and efferent signals passing along the vagus nerves, and by short intramural nervous reflexes. There is little release of gastrin, as measured by radioimmunoassay of the hormone in blood, when the whole stomach is distended. On the other hand, experimental distention of the gastric antrum enhances gastric secretion both by the release of gastrin and by local neural mechanisms.

In physiologic terms, neural mechanisms are of primary importance in the gastric secretory response to distention of the stomach by a meal. However, it is gastrin which is responsible for the secretory effect of specific chemical stimulants in a meal. The partial digestion products of proteins (i.e., polypeptides, smaller protein fragments, and amino acids) are potent stimulants of gastrin release. Of the amino acids, phenylalanine and tryptophan appear to be particularly potent. Intact proteins do not cause this effect; thus, the proteolytic activity of basal and cephalic phase-stimulated gastric juice is important in generating the digestion products necessary for gastrin release. Calcium is another powerful intraluminal stimulant for gastrin release. Two other food items, ethanol and coffee, are stimulants of gastric secretion. The mechanisms by which these stimulants act are not fully understood.

In the small intestine, both distention and the digestion products of protein stimulate gastric secretion. At least part of the response in the *intestinal phase* is humoral. The name entero-oxyntin has been given to the hormone responsible for this phenomenon.

The stimulating mechanisms which mediate the three phases of gastric secretion are somewhat offset by inhibitory mechanisms. For example, during the cephalic phase, increased vagal activity stimulates the release of an inhibitory agent from the distal stomach and duodenum. In the stomach, acidification of the antrum to values below pH 3 inhibits the gastrin release induced by protein digestion products or antral distention. Certain important inhibitory mechanisms belong to the intestinal phase: the stimuli are acid, fat, and hyperosmolar solutions. Hydrochloric acid in the upper small intestine causes the release of secretin and a duodenal hormone called bulbogastrone, both of which depress parietal cell secretion. Dietary triglyceride must be hydrolyzed to monoglycerides and fatty acids to exert its powerful inhibitory action on gastric secretion. The fatty acids must be of chain length greater than 10 carbon atoms. Fats probably utilize a neural mechanism for inhibiting gastric secretion. There is some evidence that gastric inhibitory polypeptide (GIP) and neurotensin may also be involved. Hyperosmolar solutions in the upper small intestine depress gastric secretion, an effect which appears to involve both neural and humoral mechanisms.

Table 4–3 summarizes the stimulatory and inhibitory factors during the three phases of gastric secretion.

GASTRIC MOTILITY

The muscle layer of the stomach has three components: (1) an outer longitudinal layer, which is incomplete on the anterior and posterior surface of

TABLE 4–3. Major Components of the Three Phases of Gastric Secretion

Phase	Stimulation (+) Stimulus	Mechanism	Inhibition (−) Stimulus	Mechanism
Cephalic	Olfactory/gustatory stimuli	Vagus nerve (direct action on parietal cell and indirect via gastrin release)	Olfactory/gustatory stimuli	Vagal release of an inhibitory agent from distal stomach and duodenum
	Conditioned reflexes			
Gastric	Distention (whole stomach)	Vagus nerve	Acidification of gastric antrum	Depression of gastrin release
	Distention (antrum)	Gastrin and local neural reflexes		
	Protein digestion products, Ca^{++}	Gastrin		
	Ethanol	?		
	Coffee	?		
Intestinal	Distention	Entero-oxyntin	Acidification of upper small intestine	Secretin, bulbogastrone
	Protein digestion	Unknown mechanism(s)	Fatty acids and monoglycerides Hyperosmolar solutions	Neural reflexes, GIP, neurotensin ? Neural or humoral mechanisms

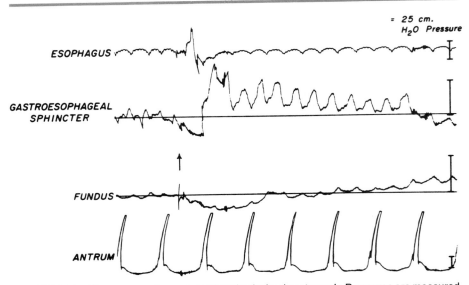

FIGURE 4–7. Time course of receptive relaxation in the dog stomach. Pressures are measured in the esophagus, gastroesophageal sphincter, and gastric fundus and antrum. Note that the fundus relaxes immediately after swallowing (at arrow). (Modified from Lind, J.F., Duthie, H.L., Schlegel, J.F., and Code, C.F.: Motility of the gastric fundus. Am. J. Physiol., *201*:197, 1961.)

the stomach, (2) a well developed (and complete) middle circular layer, and (3) an inner oblique layer, which lies on the anterior and posterior surfaces and fuses with the circular layer in the distal stomach. Intrinsic nerve plexuses are found in the wall of the stomach, the most prominent being the myenteric plexus, which lies between the longitudinal and circular muscles. Extrinsic nerves make synaptic connections with these intrinsic plexuses. The extrinsic nerve supply comes from both divisions of the autonomic nervous system; cholinergic stimulatory fibers and adrenergic and nonadrenergic inhibitory fibers have been identified.

There are three main physiologic aspects of gastric motility: (1) adaptive relaxation to accommodate a meal with a relatively small rise in intraluminal pressure, (2) contractile activity, which is responsible for thorough mixing of food with gastric juice and reducing particle size, and (3) controlled gastric emptying. In general, the proximal half of the stomach has little contractile activity and is chiefly involved in food storage (receptive relaxation), while the distal stomach is the site of vigorous contractions, especially in the postprandial state.

Figure 4–7 illustrates the time course of receptive relaxation in the dog stomach. It can be seen that relaxation of the fundus of the stomach commences with the initiation of swallowing. Even before the bolus arrives in the stomach, intragastric pressure is already reduced and, with its arrival, only small pressure changes are detected with moderate increases in volume (Fig. 4–8). For ex-

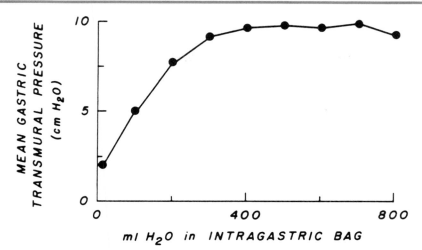

FIGURE 4–8. Pressure in the canine stomach in response to distention. (From Kelly, K.A.: Gastric motility after gastric operations. Surg. Annu., 6:103, 1974.)

ample, 225 ml of water will raise the pressure in the human stomach by less than 2 mm Hg. Afferent impulses from the mouth and esophagus are relayed via the hypothalamus to the vagal nucleus and efferent vagal inhibitory neurons are responsible for the relaxation. Hormones may also contribute, since both gastrin and cholecystokinin increase gastric distensibility, although only the action of cholecystokinin is likely to be physiologic.

While the proximal part of the stomach shows only low amplitude tonic pressure changes lasting a minute or longer, the distal stomach can show strong contractile activity after a meal (see Fig. 4–7). The proximal stomach, after receptive relaxation to accommodate a meal, gradually presses the food toward the distal stomach through sustained contractions. When contractions are present in the distal stomach, they take the form of propagated peristaltic waves occurring about three times per minute in the human stomach and four to five times per minute in the dog stomach. The peristaltic waves originate in the middle of the body of the stomach and sweep distally, gathering speed as they pass through the antrum to the pylorus. Underlying this peristaltic activity are the "pace-setter" potentials or basal electrical rhythm ($\sim$ 3 cycles/min) of the gastric smooth muscle cells. These depolarizations and repolarizations can be recorded from the midportion of the stomach and distally, but not in the proximal part. These cycles of depolarization do not necessarily result in contraction. Only when a threshold value of depolarization is exceeded and action potentials are generated does a slow wave result in a peristaltic contraction. Slow waves do not occur simultaneously throughout the stomach but are "staggered," giving a direction to the peristaltic wave such that it is propagated distally in the stomach. As recordings are taken nearer and nearer the pylorus, this lag between slow waves at successive points along the long axis of the

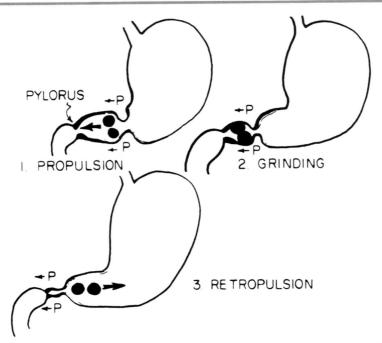

FIGURE 4–9. Consequences of antral peristalsis. (From Kelly, K.A. *In* Johnson, L.R. (ed.): Physiology of the Gastrointestinal Tract. New York, Raven Press, 1981, p. 400.)

stomach becomes shorter; thus, the contractile wave gathers speed as it approaches the pylorus.

The contractile activity of the distal stomach is influenced by both neural and humoral factors. Vagal cholinergic efferent fibers enhance the contractions while other vagal efferents and sympathetic fibers inhibit them. The afferents which initiate these efferent impulses include stretch and pH-sensitive nerve fibers in the stomach wall. Gastrin increases the frequency of the pace-setter potentials by about one cycle per minute and stimulates the appearance of action potentials, thereby increasing both the occurrence and frequency of contractions.

Peristaltic contractions of the distal stomach propel the gastric contents toward the pylorus. Liquids in the chyme are allowed to pass through the pylorus but solids are retained. As the contractions reach the terminal antrum, the pylorus closes, and solids are ground in this "mill." Since the material cannot pass forward, it is retropelled into the body of the stomach (Fig. 4–9). This retropulsion achieves very effective mixing, and the shearing forces help to disperse oil droplets as very fine emulsion particles. Until digestible solids are ground to particle sizes of less than about 0.2 mm, they are retained in the stomach. Antral contractions are relatively unimportant in terms of transferring fluid from the stomach to the duodenum.

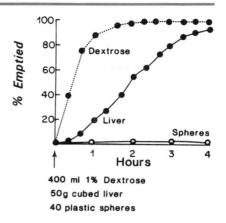

FIGURE 4–10. Patterns of canine gastric emptying of a liquid, a digestible solid, and an indigestible solid after their concurrent ingestion. (From Hinder, R.A., and Kelly, K.A.: Canine gastric emptying of solids and liquids. Am. J. Physiol., *233*:E335, 1977.)

The pylorus is a thickened band of the circular muscle layer. Although called a sphincter, there is little evidence that it really functions as such, since there is no zone of high pressure in the pyloric ring. The pylorus appears to be responsible for impeding the entry of large solid particles into the duodenum, and its closure at the end of antral contractions promotes mixing in the stomach. Its closure during duodenal contractions prevents duodenogastric reflux and forces duodenal contents to move distally.

Gastric Emptying

Gastric emptying of liquids is not dependent on the activity of the pylorus but simply depends on the pressure gradient across it. Digestible solids, on the other hand, empty more slowly than liquids, and here the pylorus appears to play an important role. Indigestible solids leave the stomach even more slowly (Fig. 4–10). Fluids at body temperature leave the stomach more rapidly than colder or warmer solutions, and large volumes of fluid leave the stomach (measured in ml/min) faster than small volumes. Isotonic saline leaves the stomach at a rate such that the square root of the volume remaining in the stomach declines linearly with time (Fig. 4–11). In man, the half-time for saline emptying is 12 min.

The composition of chyme is the major regulator of gastric emptying (Table 4–4). Carbohydrates empty faster than proteins, which, in turn, empty faster than fats. Acid solutions empty more slowly than neutral ones, and isotonic solutions leave the stomach faster than hypo- or hypertonic solutions. Receptors localized in the mucosa of the proximal small intestine sense the pH, fatty acid content, and osmolarity of chyme. These receptors regulate gastric emptying through hormonal and neural mechanisms. Unhydrolyzed triglycerides do not activate the receptors. Fatty acids, monoglycerides, and diglycerides, however, do stimulate the receptors. It is only *long*-chain fatty acids which have this effect, and the optimal chain length is 14 carbon atoms (myristic acid). The response to stimulating the fatty acid receptor is so rapid that it is likely to

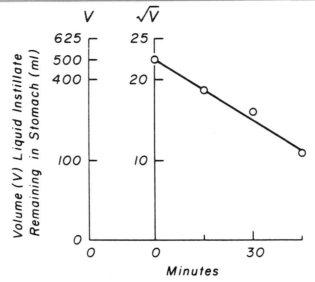

FIGURE 4–11.   Gastric emptying of 500 ml of isotonic saline in the dog. (From Kelly, K.A.: Gastric motility after gastric operations. Surg. Annu., 6:103, 1974.)

involve a neural mechanism, at least in part. Of the hormones thought to be involved, cholecystokinin and possibly neurotensin are the likely candidates.

Gastric emptying is impaired by vagotomy. The overall tone of the stomach is reduced and gastric stasis results, suggesting that a background of vagal activity is necessary for normal gastric emptying. Surgeons performing a vagotomy to reduce gastric secretion also carry out a "drainage procedure" at the same time to overcome this problem. This consists of a pyloroplasty (in which the pylorus is refashioned) or a side-to-side anastomosis between the stomach and the small intestine, a gastroenterostomy, which creates an additional exit route from the stomach.

TABLE 4–4.   Regulation of Gastric Emptying

Stimulus	Mediator	Effect on Gastric Emptying
Gastric Control		
Distention	Acetylcholine (Vago-vagal reflex)	Increase
	Gastrin	Increase
Digested protein	Gastrin	Increase
Intestinal Control		
Low duodenal pH	Secretin	Decrease
Hypertonic chyme	Hormone/Reflex	Decrease
Fat digestion	Cholecystokinin Neurotensin GIP	Decrease
L-tryptophan	Cholecystokinin	Decrease
Distention or irritation of duodenum	Vago-vagal and local inhibitory fibers	Decrease

OVERVIEW OF THE GASTRIC RESPONSE TO A MEAL

With the preceding information, together with data from direct studies in man, it is possible to construct a scheme of events in the stomach when a meal is taken and for the hours that follow.

In the fasting state, the human stomach contains only a small amount of swallowed air, 20 to 30 ml of gastric secretion, saliva, and debris. Some refluxed duodenal secretion is also often present. The pH of the gastric content is low, generally between 1 and 2. Regarding motor activity, the stomach oscillates between quiescence and activity during fasting (the interdigestive pattern of motor activity). Cycles of activity occur every 1 to 2 hours. These cycles involve periods of irregular contraction lasting about 15 to 45 minutes followed by periods of intense rhythmic activity lasting about 5 minutes.

From the start of a meal, gastric secretion increases and may even precede eating if there is a pronounced psychic component (anticipation) in the cephalic phase. Secretion accelerates and subsequently decelerates, the peak being reached at 30 to 60 minutes (Fig. 4–12). One can infer that during the accelerating phase, the positive factors controlling gastric secretion (see Table 4–3) predominate, while inhibitory factors are more important in the decelerating phase. The arrival of food in the stomach quickly raises the pH owing to dilution and buffering of gastric acid. The cephalic phase in man, accounting for 30 to 40 per cent of maximal secretory capacity, is reinforced by gastric distention as food arrives in the stomach. This accounts for an additional 30 per cent of the maximal secretory response to a meal. The final 30 per cent is provided by chemical release of gastrin. It is likely that intestinal factors are responsible for only a minor proportion of the gastric secretory response. Since chyme enters the small intestine very shortly after a meal has been ingested, the small intestine may exert its stimulating effect quite early in the postprandial period.

The decline in gastric secretion following a meal is due, to a large extent, to acidification of gastric contents. This is the result of continuous acid secretion, which eventually overcomes the buffering effect of the food. When gastric pH falls to about 2, acid secretion declines owing to inhibition of antral gastrin release. It is likely that the remainder of the inhibition is due to mechanisms activated by acid, fat, and carbohydrate entering the small intestine. As illustrated in Figure 4–12, gastric secretion rate returns to its basal level within two hours from the start of a meal.

Shortly after food enters the stomach, vigorous antral contractions occur with intraluminal pressures rising as high as 100 mm Hg. The frequency and force of the antral contractions gradually decline after the first postprandial hour and the pattern of gastric motility during fasting begins to re-establish itself.

During their residence in the stomach, foodstuffs undergo limited enzymatic hydrolysis. Starch digestion by salivary amylase can continue to some extent but as acidity increases, this activity declines. Lipolysis, however, can continue to a moderate extent, since oral lipase can function at acid pH. Thus

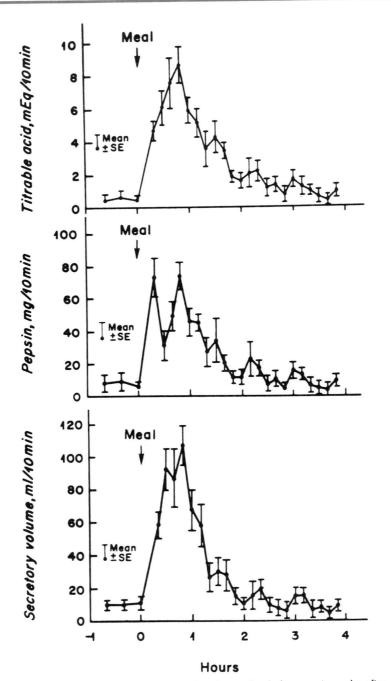

FIGURE 4–12.   Outputs of acid, pepsin, and total secretion in human stomachs after a meal. (From Malagelada, J.R.: Gastroenterology, *78*:826, 1980.)

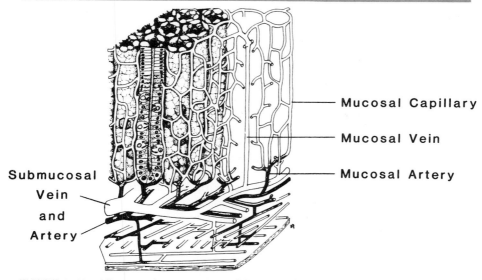

Mucosal Capillary

Mucosal Vein

Submucosal Vein and Artery

Mucosal Artery

FIGURE 4–13. Microvascular organization of the stomach. (Modified from Ohtani, O., Kikuta, A., Ohtsuka, A., Taguchi, T., and Murakami, T.: Microvasculature as studied by the microvascular corrosion casting/scanning electron microscope method. I. Endocrine and digestive system. Arch. Histol. Jpn., *46*:1–42, 1983.)

some free fatty acid is released. Short-chain fatty acids liberated from milk triglycerides can be absorbed and transported in the gastric venous blood. Released long-chain fatty acids probably help to stabilize the coarse emulsion of dietary fats. Proteins also play a role in stabilizing the fat emulsion. Retropulsion of gastric content as a result of antral activity provides energy for creating the emulsion. The fatty acids of chyme are also important because, on entering the small intestine, they play a role in regulating gastric emptying. Peptic proteolysis provides the peptides, which stimulate gastrin release, and the amino acids, which stimulate cholecystokinin release in the small intestine.

Gastric emptying begins shortly after food enters the stomach. If water is ingested with a solid meal, it leaves the stomach quite rapidly while the solids remain behind. Gastric secretion replaces the water, thus allowing continued digestion and reduction of particle size by the antral mill. Digestible solids are ground very finely. Nondigestible solids are retained until very late in the postprandial period. If solids cannot be greatly reduced in size, they tend to leave the stomach as the interdigestive pattern of motor activity returns. The time frame of emptying of a mixed meal, i.e., approximately four hours, is to a large extent determined by its chemical composition, notably its fat content.

GASTRIC BLOOD FLOW

Figure 4–13 is a diagrammatic representation of the arrangement of the blood vessels in each layer of the stomach wall. The arteries, as they pierce the muscle layer, give off branches to the musculature which ultimately break up into a capillary network. In the submucosa, arterial plexuses are found, from which arterioles supplying the mucosa pass perpendicularly through the muscularis mucosae. The tone of the submucosal arterioles determines the magnitude of the mucosal blood flow. The venous drainage of the stomach layers can be seen to follow a pattern similar to that of the arterial supply. It is estimated that approximately 70 per cent of gastric blood flow goes to the mucosa and, at high rates of flow, this proportion may be even higher.

Gastric blood flow is controlled by neural, humoral, and metabolic factors. Sympathetic nervous activity reduces total gastric blood flow and mucosal flow through arteriolar constriction. Sustained sympathetic stimulation leads to an escape from this constriction ("autoregulatory escape") due to relaxation of initially constricted vessels. The vagus, on the other hand, appears to send direct vasodilator fibers to gastric vessels, and vagotomy, at least in the short term (over a few months), reduces gastric mucosal blood flow, suggesting a tonic vasodilator influence of the parasympathetic nervous supply.

Several hormones and histamine are known to influence gastric blood flow. For example, gastrin enhances mucosal blood flow, but whether this enhancement is a direct action on blood vessels or is linked with its secretagogue action is not clear. Histamine is a vasodilator of the gastric circulation; there appear to be both H_1 and H_2 receptors in gastric submucosal arterioles which respond to histamine by dilatation. Somatostatin, a peptide found in endocrine-type cells in the stomach, pancreas, and intestine, reduces gastric blood flow as does the posterior pituitary peptide, vasopressin. These latter two agents have been used clinically to help arrest acute upper gastrointestinal bleeding.

Elaboration of gastric juice requires metabolic energy. This is demonstrated by the observation that oxygen consumption by the stomach increases in proportion to acid production. At high rates of blood flow, the oxygen supply for secretion is easily met by the tissue extracting the requisite amount of oxygen from the blood. Thus, there is no correlation between blood flows and acid production at high blood flows. At low blood flows, however, acid secretion and blood flow fall in parallel, owing to the fact that at these low flows the rate of oxygen delivery to the parietal cells is limited by blood flow.

Gastric venous blood normally drains into the portal vein. Thus, substances absorbed from the stomach such as water, ethanol, and a proportion of water- and lipid-soluble nutrients are delivered to the liver by this route. When portal venous pressure is chronically elevated, as occurs for example in cirrhosis of the liver, the gastric venous circulation drains partly into the systemic circulation through anastomotic veins which open up in the distal esophagus and empty into the azygos system. These dilated veins, termed esophageal varices, partly decompress the hypertensive portal venous system. They are, however, prone to sudden rupture with severe upper gastrointestinal hemorrhage.

GASTRIC MUCOSAL BARRIER

How does the gastric mucosa protect itself against its own secreted acid? In common with certain other tissues of the digestive tract, the stomach faces

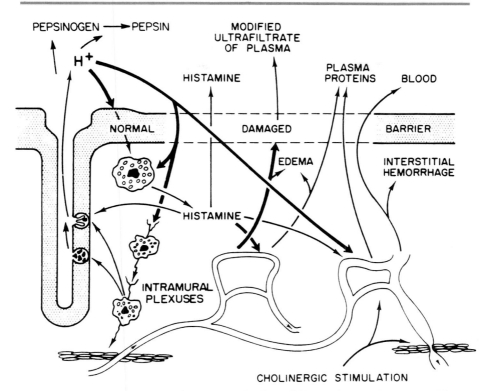

FIGURE 4–14. Effects of excessive "back diffusion" of H+ on the gastric mucosa. (From Davenport, H.W.: Physiology of the Digestive Tract. Chicago, Year Book Medical Publishers, 1977, p. 124.)

the problem that its own secretions are potentially injurious. Agents such as pancreatic enzymes and bile salts can also damage epithelial membranes. If hydrogen ions do penetrate the mucosal membrane in large amounts, their presence in the interstitium of the mucosa leads to vasodilatation, edema, epithelial cell necrosis and sloughing, and mucosal hemorrhage (Fig. 4–14). Local release of histamine may be involved in this process. Such damage to the mucosal membrane leads to the escape of interstitial fluid and plasma proteins into the gastric lumen and, with severe damage, blood cells will be released.

When the mucosal membrane is broken, the high concentration gradient of H+ across the gastric mucosa favors "back diffusion" of acid. That this does not happen to any great degree normally, is the result of the resistance of the mucosal epithelial layer to such diffusion and is termed the "gastric mucosal barrier." This barrier represents the healthy functioning of the surface mucous cells, the integrity of their tight intercellular junctions, and their covering layer of mucus trapping an alkaline fluid. An adequate mucosal blood flow is important, presumably because it preserves the normal metabolic functions of the surface epithelium.

Certain exogenous and endogenous agents are capable of disrupting the barrier and initiating the process in Figure 4–14. Bile salts and lysolecithin belong to the endogenous group. Lysolecithin, mostly derived from biliary lecithin, is a water-soluble substance with powerful detergent properties. Bile salts, similarly, are biological detergents which can solubilize membrane lipids, thereby altering the permeability characteristics of cells. Normally, the access of bile salts and lysolecithin from the small intestine to the stomach is greatly limited by the barrier to duodenal-gastric reflux at the pylorus. However, various forms of gastric surgery may destroy the antireflux mechanism with resulting "bile gastritis."

Of the exogenous substances breaking the barrier and allowing access of H^+ to the mucosa, ethanol and salicylates are the best examples. Ethanol, being lipid-soluble, can readily diffuse into the mucosa, where it interferes with enzymic processes in the epithelial cells and renders the barrier more permeable. Salicylates in acid solution exist in the un-ionized form and are lipid-soluble, diffusing readily into the mucosa. Only limited amounts of ionized salicylate can gain access to the epithelial cells. In the cell, at pH close to 7, the salicylates ionize and exert toxic effects on cell metabolism, causing enhanced permeability to H^+. The combination of ethanol and salicylate, in the presence of acid, is particularly potent in disrupting the gastric mucosal barrier. It is not unusual to encounter patients with hemorrhagic gastritis resulting from the use of aspirin to relieve the "hangover" of excessive alcohol intake.

VOMITING

Vomiting, or forceful expulsion of gastric contents, should be distinguished from both regurgitation resulting from a lax lower esophageal sphincter in infants and esophageal reflux in adults. It is usual that, before vomiting, the nauseated person retches. This involves closure of the glottis following deep inspiration. Strong contractions of the abdominal muscles raise intra-abdominal pressure, creating a large pressure gradient between abdomen and thorax. The antrum contracts, directing gastric content to the body of the stomach, and a ring of contraction virtually divides the contracted antrum from the flaccid body of the stomach. The intra-abdominal pressure forces the abdominal part of the esophagus and cardiac portion of the stomach briefly into the thorax. Then, the gastric contents are forced into the esophagus, which is dilated and has no peristaltic activity at the time. Since the pharyngoesophageal sphincter is closed, nothing is expelled into the pharynx. The abdominal muscles then relax, and the esophageal contents return to the stomach. The cycle is repeated a number of times.

Vomiting is the extension of the retching process. With vomiting, the abdominal contractions are so strong as to force the diaphragm up into the

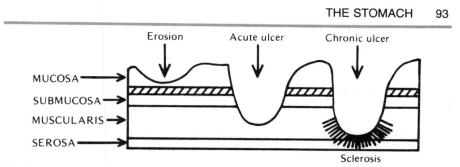

FIGURE 4–15. Diagrammatic illustration of acute and chronic gastric mucosal lesions. (From Brooks, F.P. (ed.): Gastrointestinal Pathophysiology. New York, Oxford University Press, 1978, p. 101.)

thorax, thus raising intrathoracic pressure. The larynx and hyoid bone are drawn forward. The raised intrathoracic pressure overcomes resistance from the pharyngoesophageal sphincter, and the gastric contents are expelled. Esophageal peristalsis resumes and clears what remains in the esophagus. Additional cycles may be necessary to evacuate the stomach completely, after which abdominal muscle contractions cease, and normal respiration ensues.

PAIN SENSATIONS FROM THE STOMACH

Most people suffer periodically from pain in the epigastrium, often referring to it as "indigestion." The stomach is very commonly the source of the pain, which usually results from excessive tension in the gastric wall. The afferent fibers carrying this pain sensation travel with the sympathetic nerves. Cutting or eroding the mucosa is not painful, but crushing either muscle or mucosa is.

The pain of peptic ulcer is poorly understood. Prompt neutralization of gastric acid relieves pain, and it has been suggested that acid irritating free nerve endings in the ulcer walls and base is responsible for the pain. The inflammatory tissue, however, insulates the nerve endings from gastric juice. It is possible that local muscle spasm is the primary cause of ulcer pain.

CLINICAL CORRELATIONS

Acid-Peptic Disease

This group of conditions accounts for a major proportion of gastrointestinal diseases. These diseases range from inflammation and superficial ulcerations and erosions of the mucosa to chronic ulceration, which may penetrate to a considerable depth in the gut wall (Fig. 4–15). The esophagus, stomach, and duodenum are affected. Peptic esophagitis results from a failure of the lower esophageal sphincter to prevent access of gastric juice to the distal esophagus.

An incompetent lower esophageal sphincter allows reflux of gastric juice, particularly when the person is in the recumbent position. Inflammation and superficial ulceration of the distal esophageal mucosa cause pain on swallowing (odynophagia), and chronic peptic esophagitis can lead to cicatrization (scarring) of the distal esophagus with strictures that impede the passage of the food bolus.

In the stomach and duodenum, similar inflammation, erosions, and ulceration can cause pain and periodic bleeding. Ulcers can extend through the full thickness of the gut wall and either perforate, allowing the escape of gastroduodenal fluids into the peritoneal cavity, or penetrate into neighboring organs, notably the pancreas. Two factors operate in the pathologic process: the aggressive actions of HCl and pepsin, and the resistance of the mucosa to this attack. It is generally believed that in the esophagus and duodenum the aggressive factors are more important but in acid-peptic disease of the stomach impaired mucosal resistance may be of considerable importance. An example of the aggressive action of gastric juice occurs in the rare gastrinoma syndrome, in which uncontrolled hypersecretion of gastrin from an endocrine tumor occurs. Gastric acid output is often greatly elevated, as a result of both excessive stimulation of the parietal cells and an expanded parietal cell mass resulting from gastrin's trophic action on the parietal cells. Normally, the duodenum efficiently titrates gastric acid with alkaline secretions, i.e., bile, pancreatic juice, and Brunner's gland secretions. Duodenal pH is generally between 6 and 7 but, in the gastrinoma syndrome, the neutralization process can be overwhelmed, leading to severe duodenal ulceration and even ulceration as far distal as the jejunum.

Peptic ulceration does not occur in the absence of gastric acid, i.e., achlorhydria; patients with Addisonian pernicious anemia, an autoimmune process which destroys the parietal cells, do not develop ulcers. The serum gastrin concentration in these patients is elevated, since they never acidify the antrum; thus, there is no "brake" on gastrin secretion. Since intrinsic factor is derived from parietal cells, these patients develop megaloblastic anemia due to malabsorption of vitamin B_{12}.

The mainstay of treatment of acid-peptic disease has been to remove or inactivate acid and pepsin, allowing the gastroduodenal mucosa to regenerate and repair itself. Traditional treatment has been the neutralization of gastric acid and the inactivation of pepsin by antacids such as aluminum and magnesium hydroxides. Section of the entire vagus nerve, or its gastric branches, permanently reduces the magnitude of the gastric secretory response. Pharmacologic approaches have included antisecretory agents such as anticholinergic drugs and, more recently, selective H_2 receptor antihistamines such as cimetidine and ranitidine. Future developments may involve methods of improving the tissue resistance to the attack of acid and pepsin. Prostaglandins, which appear to afford protection to mucosal cells against acid-pepsin attack, termed "cytoprotection," hold some promise in this connection.

Metabolic Disturbances Due to Loss of Gastric Secretion

Gastric outlet obstruction can lead to vomiting with excessive loss of gastric secretions. This loss can also result from prolonged nasogastric suction. From a consideration of the composition of gastric juice, it can be seen that the losses will include water, H^+, Na^+, K^+ and Cl^-, with the major metabolic disturbances being dehydration and hypokalemic alkalosis. This alkalosis is perpetuated by contraction of the extracellular fluid volume due to water and sodium chloride loss in gastric juice and the development of potassium deficiency due to secondary aldosteronism and the loss of K^+ in the gastric juice. Since the renal compensatory mechanisms do not correct this complex disturbance, careful fluid and electrolyte replacement is necessary in such patients.

REFERENCES

Davenport, H.W.: Physiology of the Digestive Tract. Chicago, Year Book Medical Publishers, 1977.

Fromm, D.: Gastric mucosal barrier. In Johnson, L.R. (ed.): Physiology of the Gastrointestinal Tract. New York, Raven Press, 1981, pp. 733–748.

Grossman, M.I.: Regulation of gastric acid secretion. In Johnson, L.R. (ed.): Physiology of the Gastrointestinal Tract. New York, Raven Press, 1981, pp. 659–671.

Ito, S.: Functional gastric morphology. In Johnson, L.R. (ed.): Physiology of the Gastrointestinal Tract. New York, Raven Press, 1981, pp. 517–550.

Kelly, K.A.: Motility of the stomach and gastroduodenal junction. In Johnson, L.R. (ed.): Physiology of the Gastrointestinal Tract. New York, Raven Press, 1981, pp. 393–410.

Malagelada, J.R.: Gastric, pancreatic and biliary responses to a meal. In Johnson, L.R. (ed.): Physiology of the Gastrointestinal Tract. New York, Raven Press, 1981, pp. 893–924.

Minami, H., and McCallum, R.W.: The physiology and pathophysiology of gastric emptying in humans. Gastroenterology, 86:1592–1610, 1984.

The pancreas is both an exocrine and an endocrine organ. The endocrine activity of the pancreas is localized in clusters of specialized cells (islets of Langerhans) interspersed throughout the gland. The islet cells, which comprise only 2 to 3 per cent of the parenchyma, secrete several important hormones of which insulin, glucagon, and somatostatin are the most notable examples. The exocrine pancreas elaborates a secretion which is delivered to the duodenum, where it plays an important role in the digestive process. This exocrine secretion, termed pancreatic juice, contains two functionally important constituents: bicarbonate ions and digestive enzymes. The bicarbonate ions neutralize the acidic chyme entering the duodenum from the stomach. Raising the pH of chyme not only protects the mucosal epithelia from injury, but also provides an optimal pH for the activity of the pancreatic enzymes. The digestive enzymes of the juice are capable of degrading all of the major nutrients of ingested food, i.e., carbohydrates, proteins, and lipids. Although the contribution of the pancreas to the digestive process has traditionally been attributed solely to its exocrine functions, it is becoming increasingly apparent that the hormones secreted by the islet cells can modulate the rate of formation and the composition of pancreatic juice.

5

THE PANCREAS

ANATOMY

The pancreas, situated in close apposition to the duodenum, is a compound acinous gland whose lobules are bound together by loose connective tissue. The lobules are composed of clusters of acini which are structurally similar to those of the serous salivary glands. The acinus consists of six to eight pyramidally shaped acinar cells (with their apices facing the lumen) and a few irregularly shaped centroacinar cells (Fig. 5–1). The acinar cells are specialized for protein secretion and contain an elaborate network of rough endoplasmic reticulum in the basal portion of the cell, a Golgi complex in the midportion, and numerous zymogen granules in the apical region. The centroacinar cells, which are the initial components of the duct system, are characterized by a sparse cytoplasm devoid of zymogen granules but containing many large mitochondria. The centroacinar cells and the cuboidal cells of the intercalated duct, which drains the acinus, appear to be the primary sites of electrolyte and water secretion.

The intercalated ducts converge to form intralobular ducts, which, in turn,

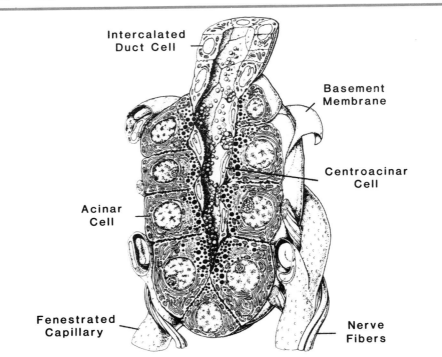

Intercalated
Duct Cell

Basement
Membrane

Centroacinar
Cell

Acinar
Cell

Fenestrated
Capillary

Nerve
Fibers

FIGURE 5–1. The pancreatic acinus. × 3000. (Adapted from Johnson, L.R.: Physiology of the Digestive Tract. New York, Raven Press, 1981, p. 796.)

drain into interlobular ducts. The interlobular ducts empty their contents into one of two main ducts that deliver the secretion to the duodenum. The major pancreatic duct (duct of Wirsung) enters the duodenum at the ampulla of Vater alongside the common bile duct, both being surrounded by a ring of smooth muscle called the sphincter of Oddi. In some individuals (< 40 per cent), the major pancreatic duct and the common bile duct join before entering the duodenum. The minor duct (duct of Santorini) enters the duodenum a few centimeters cephalad to the sphincter of Oddi. In 70 to 90 per cent of individuals, the two pancreatic ducts are in structural continuity within the gland.

Regulation of Pancreatic Mass

It is well recognized that starvation or parenteral feeding results in pancreatic atrophy. Cholecystokinin, a hormone released from the intestinal mucosa in response to luminal nutrients, is considered to be a major regulator of pancreatic growth. Exogenous administration of cholecystokinin (CCK) to experimental animals results in pancreatic growth. Furthermore, pancreatic growth can result from feeding soybean trypsin inhibitor, which stimulates the release of CCK.

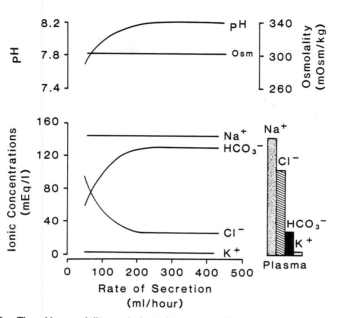

FIGURE 5–2. The pH, osmolality, and electrolyte composition of pancreatic juice at different rates of secretion. Plasma levels of electrolytes are given for reference.

COMPOSITION OF PANCREATIC JUICE

The human pancreas can secrete roughly one liter of pancreatic juice (equivalent to ten times its weight) per day. The secreted juice contains a variety of electrolytes and proteins, the concentrations of which vary with the mode of stimulation. The principal anions are Cl^- and HCO_3^- and the principal cations are Na^+ and K^+. Pancreatic enzymes account for more than 90 per cent of the proteins in the juice. The electrolytes and enzymes are secreted primarily by the ductular and acinar cells, respectively. Therefore, the final composition of the juice is dependent on the relative secretory activities of the ductules and acini.

Electrolytes

In contrast to saliva, pancreatic juice is isotonic with plasma at all rates of secretion (Fig. 5–2). The most likely explanation for this phenomenon is that water moves freely across pancreatic epithelia when an osmotic gradient is generated by active transport of solutes, primarily electrolytes (see Fig. 1–13 for discussion of standing osmotic gradient theory). The sum of the concentrations of cations equals that of the anions in the secreted juice and this balance is maintained at all rates of secretion. Although the Na^+ and K^+ concentrations of pancreatic juice are not affected by secretion rate, the concentrations of the major anions, HCO_3^- and Cl^-, vary dramatically with the rate of secretion. At low secretion rates, the bicarbonate concentration is equal to that of plasma, but it increases as secretion rate is stimulated by administration of secretin. The rise in HCO_3^- concentration is asymptotic, reaching a maximum value characteristic of a given species. In man, the maximum bicarbonate concentration achieved in pancreatic juice is about 130 to 140 mEq per liter, corresponding to a pH of 8.2. The relationship between Cl^- concentration in the juice and the rate of fluid secretion is the mirror image of that observed for bicarbonate. This reciprocal relationship between the concentrations of Cl^- and HCO_3^- ions is such that the sum of the two anions remains the same ($\sim$ 150 mEq per liter) regardless of the rate of secretion.

Two theories have been proposed to explain the concentration profile of the two major anions of pancreatic juice. One theory, the "anion exchange" hypothesis, is analogous to that proposed to explain electrolyte concentrations in saliva. In this scheme, the primary secretion contains a high concentration of bicarbonate and, as it moves along the ductal system, bicarbonate is exchanged for chloride. Thus, at a low flow rate, there is sufficient time for exchange to occur, and the juice contains a high concentration of Cl^- and low concentration of HCO_3^-. High rates of flow through the ducts preclude such an exchange owing to the brief contact time between the juice and ductal epithelium. On the other hand, the "two component" theory holds that one cell type (probably the acinar or centroacinar cells) secretes a fluid with plasma-like Cl^- and HCO_3^- concentrations, and that another cell type, the ductal cells, secrete a fluid rich in HCO_3^- and poor in Cl^-. At high flow rates the HCO_3^--rich ductular secretion predominates. Present evidence suggests that both mechanisms contribute to the observed pattern of electrolytes at varying secretion rates (Fig. 5–3).

The most striking feature of the electrolyte composition of pancreatic juice is the high concentration of bicarbonate at high flow rates. The mechanism of bicarbonate secretion is not completely understood, but it is generally believed that the primary event is not the active transport of HCO_3^- into the lumen but rather the active transport of H^+ out of the duct lumen (Fig. 5–4). The hydrogen entering the duct cell is exchanged for Na^+, a process requiring energy in the form of ATP. Hydrogen ions are transported out of the cell at the basal membrane in exchange for sodium. The hydrogen ions entering plasma react with bicarbonate ions to form carbon dioxide and water. The carbon dioxide generated in plasma enters the cell and, along with metabolically derived CO_2, diffuses into the ducts, where it reacts with water and the enzyme carbonic anhydrase to form hydrogen and bicarbonate ions. The bicarbonate ion then remains in the pancreatic juice, while the hydrogen ion is shuttled to plasma via the sodium-hydrogen exchange systems. This mechanism of bicarbonate secretion allows for a steady flow of hydrogen ions from duct lumen to plasma for the formation of carbon dioxide, which, in turn, is the major source (95 per

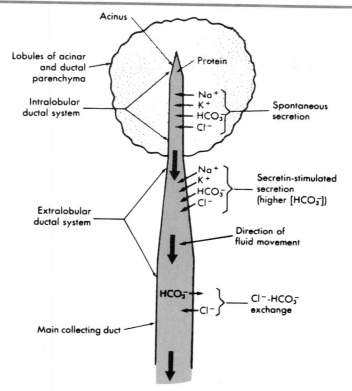

FIGURE 5–3.   The transport processes involved in the formation of pancreatic juice. (Adapted from Berne, R.M., and Levy, M.N.: Physiology. St. Louis, C.V. Mosby, 1983, p. 783.)

cent) of the bicarbonate in pancreatic juice. Chloride, the other major anion of pancreatic juice, moves passively from plasma to lumen.

Trace amounts (< 3 mEq per liter) of several other ionic species are present in pancreatic juice. These include calcium, magnesium, zinc, inorganic phosphate, and sulfate. Many stimulants of acinar cell (enzyme) secretion (e.g., vagal stimulation, cholecystokinin) also enhance the secretion of divalent cations. The concentrations of calcium and magnesium in the secreted juice are less than that of plasma. The divalent cations enter the juice by simple diffusion through paracellular pathways. As the rate of pancreatic secretion increases, the concentrations of Ca^{++} and Mg^{++} in the juice decrease. In addition to the paracellular route, calcium is released along with the enzymes contained in the zymogen granules of acinar cells. Calcium secretion during stimulation of enzyme release parallels the protein concentration in the juice and is independent of plasma levels of calcium.

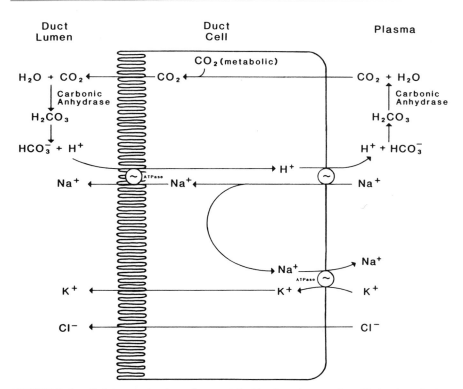

Duct
Lumen

Duct
Cell

Plasma

CO_2 (metabolic)

$H_2O + CO_2$ ← CO_2 ← $CO_2 + H_2O$

Carbonic
Anhydrase

Carbonic
Anhydrase

H_2CO_3 H_2CO_3

$HCO_3^- + H^+$ $H^+ + HCO_3^-$

H^+

Na^+ ← Na^+ Na^+

Na^+ Na^+

K^+ ← K^+ ← K^+

Cl^- ← Cl^-

FIGURE 5–4. Cellular mechanism of pancreatic bicarbonate secretion. Carbonic anhydrase is present in both red blood cells and the ductular microvilli.

Proteins

Pancreatic juice contains a variety of proteins, the majority of which (> 90 per cent) are hydrolases and can be classified according to the specific substrates upon which they act (Table 5–1). Most of the enzymes of pancreatic juice are proteolytic. They are synthesized, stored, and secreted as inactive precursors (called proenzymes) which are activated in the duodenal lumen. Activation of the proteases involves hydrolytic cleavage of key peptide bonds, thereby inducing a conformational change in the enzyme which unmasks the "catalytic site" or the "binding site." The initial step in duodenal activation of pancreatic proteases is accomplished by an endopeptidase secreted by the enterocytes. This peptidase (inappropriately referred to as enterokinase) converts trypsinogen to its active form, trypsin. Trypsin, in turn, activates other trypsinogen molecules and the other pancreatic proteases. Amylase, ribonuclease, and the lipolytic enzymes, except phospholipase A_2, are secreted in their active forms. Pro-phospholipase A_2, like the proteases, is activated in the duodenal lumen by trypsin.

Pancreatic juice also contains two small proteins that are not enzymes yet

TABLE 5–1. Enzymes of Pancreatic Juice

Enzymes (proenzymes)	Specific Hydrolytic Activity
Proteolytic	
a) endopeptidases	
trypsin(ogen)	peptide bonds near basic residues
chymotrypsin(ogen)	peptide bonds near aromatic or other large hydrophobic residues
(pro)elastase	peptide bonds near small hydrophobic residues
b) exopeptidases	
(pro)carboxypeptidase A	all peptide bonds at carboxyl end except those near basic residues
(pro)carboxypeptidase B	only peptide bonds at carboxyl end near basic residues
(pro)aminopeptidase*	all peptide bonds at amino end
Amylolytic	
α-amylase	internal α 1,4 glucosidic bonds of glucose polymers
Lipolytic	
lipase	ester bonds at 1- and 3-positions of triglycerides
(pro)phospholipase A_2	ester bonds at 2-position of phosphoglycerides
carboxyl ester hydrolase (cholesterol esterase)	ester bonds of water-soluble lipids; cholesterol esters
Nucleolytic	
ribonuclease	phosphodiester bonds of nucleotides in ribonucleic acid
deoxyribonuclease*	phosphodiester bonds of nucleotides in deoxyribonucleic acids

*Existence in human pancreatic juice is debated.

play an important role in regulating the activity of certain pancreatic hydrolases. One of these, trypsin inhibitor, combines with trypsin in a one-to-one ratio to produce a complex that is inactive. The presence of trypsin inhibitor in the gland serves to protect the tissue from autodigestion by the small amounts of trypsin which may become activated prematurely within the pancreas. The molar concentration of trypsin inhibitor in the juice, however, is much less than the molar concentration of trypsin and, therefore, activation of the pancreatic proteases in the duodenal lumen is not prevented. Colipase, another small polypeptide present in the secreted juice, enhances the lipolytic activity of pancreatic lipase. This cofactor prevents the bile salt–induced inhibition of lipase activity by anchoring the lipase molecule to the lipid-water interface of oil droplets. The concentration of colipase in pancreatic juice is roughly equivalent to the concentration of lipase.

A minor proportion (< 10 per cent) of the proteins in pancreatic juice does not contribute to the enzymatic functions of the juice. Immunoglobulin A (secretory type) and lactoferrin are synthesized and secreted by the pancreas. These two proteins are commonly found in most exocrine secretions (e.g., saliva, tears, milk), where they may act as antibacterial agents. Plasma proteins can also enter the juice by filtration. Albumin, the immunoglobulins A, G, and M, transferrin, and α_2-macroglobulin have thus far been identified in pancreatic juice.

The synthesis, packaging, and secretion of proteins (i.e., enzymes) is an orderly sequence of events proceeding from the basal to apical regions of the pancreatic acinar cell. The peptide chain is synthesized in the rough endoplasmic reticulum located in the basal portion of the cell, processed in the Golgi apparatus, and stored in zymogen granules at the apical region. In response to an appropriate neural or humoral stimulus or both, the zymogen granule membrane fuses with the apical cell membrane and subsequently releases the granule contents into the duct lumen.

Each zymogen granule is believed to contain the entire complement of pancreatic enzymes synthesized by the acinar cells and, therefore, the enzymes are secreted in a constant proportion when the pancreas is stimulated. Since the ratio of one enzyme to another is identical in pancreatic juice and zymogen granules, it appears that the relative concentrations of the different enzymes in the juice are determined at the time of synthesis. However, the relative concentration of the enzymes in the juice can be altered by the diet, i.e., the concentration of a given enzyme (lipase) can be increased when the level of its substrate (fat) in the diet is raised. For the most part, such adaptation of pancreatic enzyme secretion to dietary stimulants is believed to require several weeks of dietary modification before it is fully established.

REGULATION OF PANCREATIC SECRETION

Hormonal Regulation

The most potent humoral stimulants of pancreatic secretion are secretin and cholecystokinin. Secretin primarily stimulates the secretion of bicarbonate and water by the duct cells. It also exerts a mild stimulatory effect on enzyme output by the acinar cells. Conversely, cholecystokinin is a potent stimulant of enzyme secretion but a weak stimulant of fluid and bicarbonate output. Other peptides structurally related to these two agonists produce predictable effects on pancreatic secretion. Vasoactive intestinal polypeptide (VIP) is structurally similar to secretin and can stimulate bicarbonate and water secretion. VIP is a weaker agonist than secretin. When VIP is administered along with secretin it competitively inhibits the secretory effects of the latter. Gastrin possesses the same carboxy-terminal structure as cholecystokinin and can stimulate pancreatic enzyme output. The effect of gastrin is considerably less than that of cholecystokinin, and gastrin can inhibit the cholecystokinin-induced enzyme output. Because of these structure-activity relationships, pancreatic cells are believed to have both secretin and CCK receptors which recognize structural analogues of each of these hormones.

Other peptide hormones have been shown to alter pancreatic secretion by acting on receptors other than the secretin and cholecystokinin receptors. Pancreatic polypeptide, pancreatone, and somatostatin are inhibitors of pancreatic secretion, while substance P and neurotensin are pancreatic stimulants. The physiologic importance of these peptides in secretory responses is yet to be fully determined.

Neural Regulation

The parasympathetic innervation of the pancreas is derived from the dorsal vagal nucleus. Preganglionic axons emerge from the brainstem in the vagus nerve and synapse on cell bodies of postganglionic fibers within the substance of the pancreas. The intrinsic postganglionic fibers, in turn, innervate islet, ductular, and acinar cells. Acetylcholine is the neurotransmitter released near the effector cells during vagal stimulation; in some species, VIP has also been identified in the postganglionic nerve terminals. In all species studied, activation of the efferent parasympathetic (vagal) fibers or administration of acetylcholine enhances pancreatic enzyme secretion with little or no effect on bicarbonate and water output. The enzyme output in response to nerve stimulation or cholinergic agents can be abolished by atropine. In those species where a modest increase in water and bicarbonate secretion is associated with vagally mediated enzyme secretion, the bicarbonate response is not affected by atropine. The concomitant release of VIP from postganglionic fibers is probably responsible for the bicarbonate and water secretion induced by vagal stimulation.

The preganglionic sympathetic fibers supplying the pancreas orginate in the fifth to tenth thoracic segments, pass down to the level of the lower six thoracic and upper two lumbar ganglia, and synapse with postganglionic fibers in the celiac and superior mesenteric ganglia. The postganglionic fibers course with the arterial blood vessels to the gland. The postganglionic nerve terminals are in close association with vascular smooth muscle rather than the parenchyma. The neurotransmitter released at the sympathetic nerve terminal is norepinephrine. In general, stimulation of the splanchnic nerve has either no effect or inhibits pancreatic secretion. The inhibition of pancreatic secretion is believed to be secondary to the sympathetically mediated constriction of blood vessels supplying the pancreas.

Stimulus-Secretion Coupling

All agents which increase pancreatic secretion appear to exert their effects by initiating one of two distinct intracellular events, i.e., increasing intracellular concentrations of cyclic AMP or calcium (Fig. 5–5). Secretin and VIP, both potent stimulants of bicarbonate and water secretion, bind with cell membrane receptors and increase intracellular concentrations of cyclic AMP by activating adenyl cyclase. The interaction of cholecystokinin and acetylcholine with their receptors results in an increased intracellular free calcium concentration by

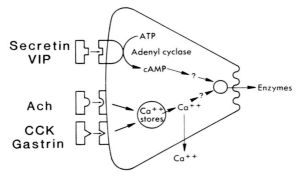

FIGURE 5–5. Intracellular mechanisms involved in stimulus-secretion coupling.

mobilizing intracellular stores. Since intracellular stores of calcium are limited, and calcium leaves the cells with the proteins (enzymes), sustained enzyme secretion in response to cholecystokinin is dependent on an intracellular influx of calcium from the plasma. The increased bicarbonate and water secretion produced by secretin is associated with hyperpolarization of the duct cells, whereas the enhanced enzyme secretion caused by cholecystokinin is associated with depolarization of the acinar cells, indicating that changes in the electrical potential of the cells may play a role in stimulus-secretion coupling.

Potentiation of Secretory Responses

Secretin can potentiate the effects of cholecystokinin on pancreatic enzyme secretion, while cholecystokinin can potentiate the effects of secretin on bicarbonate and water secretion. The magnitude of the change in pancreatic protein secretion in response to the two hormones exceeds the sum of the effects of each hormone alone. Potentiation of the bicarbonate and water responses to secretin and cholecystokinin is more dramatic than their potentiating effect on protein secretion. There are similar synergisms between secretin and gastrin and between VIP and cholecystokinin. At the cellular level, potentiation requires that the stimuli act on different membrane receptors and trigger different intracellular events, which subsequently lead to the same secretory response (Fig. 5–5). Since secretin and cholecystokinin stimulate different receptors and use different stimulus-secretion coupling mechanisms, they can potentiate each other's actions. Vagal stimulation (or acetylcholine) and cholecystokinin, which trigger identical intracellular events, are only additive.

OVERVIEW OF PANCREATIC SECRETORY RESPONSE TO MEALS (Table 5–2)

Basal Secretion

Basal pancreatic secretion of bicarbonate is 2 to 3 per cent of the maximal secretory response, while the enzymes are secreted at 10 to 15 per cent of the

TABLE 5–2. Summary of Factors Regulating Pancreatic Exocrine Secretion Postprandially

Phase of Digestion	Stimulus	Mediators	Pancreatic Response
Cephalic	Taste, smell, chewing and swallowing of food	Acetylcholine or Gastrin released by vagal impulses	Increased rate of secretion with a greater effect on enzyme output
Gastric	Gastric distention	Acetylcholine released by vagal impulses	Increased rate of secretion with a greater effect on enzyme output
	Protein in the stomach	Gastrin	Increased rate of secretion with a greater effect on enzyme output
Intestinal	Titratable acid	Secretin	Increased rate of secretion with a greater effect on bicarbonate and water output
	Fat and protein digestion products	Cholecystokinin	Increased rate of secretion with a greater effect on enzyme output
	Fat and protein digestion products	Acetylcholine released by vagal impulses	Increased rate of secretion with a greater effect on enzyme output
	Ca^{++} in the lumen of upper small intestine	Unknown	Increased rate of secretion with a greater effect on enzyme output
	Bile in the lumen of upper small intestine	Unknown	Increased rate of enzyme, bicarbonate, and water secretion
	Trypsin in the lumen of the upper small intestine	Inhibition of cholecystokinin release	Decreased rate of secretion with a greater effect on enzyme output
	Fat digestion products/hypertonic glucose in ileum or colon	Pancreatone	Decreased rate of enzyme, bicarbonate, and water secretion
	Increased blood levels of glucose and amino acids	Pancreatic hormones (somatostatin, glucagon, pancreatic polypeptide)	Decreased rate of enzyme secretion

maximal output. The stimuli responsible for basal levels of secretion are not known but may be due to the relatively low levels of circulating secretagogues and neural activity. Inasmuch as a denervated pancreas perfused with physiologic solutions devoid of hormones can secrete, basal secretion can be attributed, at least in part, to some intrinsic mechanism.

Cephalic Phase of Secretion

The cephalic phase of pancreatic secretion is initiated by the smell, taste, chewing, and swallowing of food (Fig. 5–6). The enhanced pancreatic secretion during the cephalic phase represents 10 to 15 per cent of the volume and 25

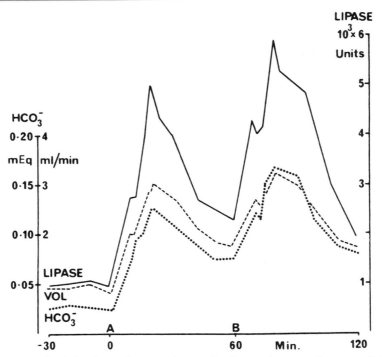

FIGURE 5–6. Cephalic phase of pancreatic secretion in man. Increases in pancreatic lipase, bicarbonate, and water output occurred in response to visual and olfactory stimuli (grilling of beefsteak) at point A, and in response to gustatory stimuli (chewing and tasting the grilled steak) at point B. (Adapted from Howat, H.T., and Sarles, H.: The Exocrine Pancreas. London, W.B. Saunders, 1979, p. 67.)

per cent of the enzyme response to a meal. Sham feeding also elicits a pancreatic secretion rich in enzymes. Both atropine and vagotomy block the enhanced secretion during the cephalic phase, indicating that the parasympathetic neurotransmitter, acetylcholine, mediates this response. Acetylcholine, released from postganglionic terminals in the pancreas, could directly stimulate duct and acinar cells to secrete a protein-rich fluid. Alternatively, acetylcholine released by postganglionic cholinergic fibers in the antrum may indirectly enhance pancreatic secretion by stimulating gastrin release.

Gastric Phase of Secretion

The gastric phase of pancreatic secretion is triggered by the entrance of food into the stomach. Distention of the stomach with a balloon results in a pancreatic secretory response similar to that observed during the cephalic phase i.e., an enzyme-rich secretion. Since vagal transection can abolish this response, a vago-vagal (cholinergic) reflex has been implicated in the response. Gastrin may also be involved in the gastric phase of pancreatic secretion, since it is

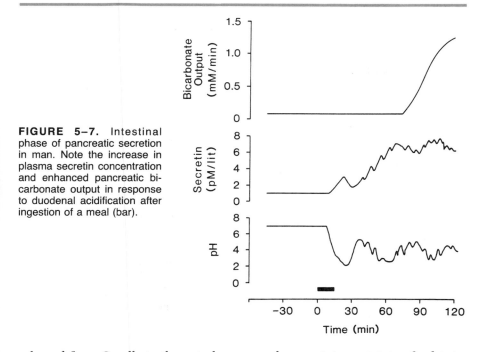

FIGURE 5–7. Intestinal phase of pancreatic secretion in man. Note the increase in plasma secretin concentration and enhanced pancreatic bicarbonate output in response to duodenal acidification after ingestion of a meal (bar).

released from G cells in the antral mucosa when protein-containing food is in the stomach.

Intestinal Phase of Secretion

The intestinal phase of pancreatic secretion is initiated by the entrance of chyme into the duodenum and accounts for 70 to 80 per cent of the pancreatic response to a meal. The acidity of the chyme and the products of protein and lipid digestion contained in chyme are the principal determinants of the type of pancreatic response elicited.

Secretin, a strong stimulant of pancreatic bicarbonate secretion, is released from the S cells in the intestinal mucosa in response to intraluminal acidity (Fig. 5–7). The increase in blood secretin concentrations is related to the degree of luminal acidity and the length of the gut exposed to acid. The threshold for secretin release is a luminal pH of about 4.5. When luminal pH falls below 4.5, the amount of secretin released is inversely related to pH, with secretin output reaching a maximum at pH 3.0. The postprandial pH of the upper small intestine rarely falls below 4.0 to 3.5 and chyme is neutralized before it enters the jejunum. Thus, the amount of secretin released after a meal is insufficient to account for the observed pancreatic bicarbonate and water secretion. This apparent discrepancy is explained by the ability of cholecystokinin and vagal impulses to potentiate the effects of small amounts of circulating secretin on the ductule cells of the pancreas. This hypothesis is supported by the finding

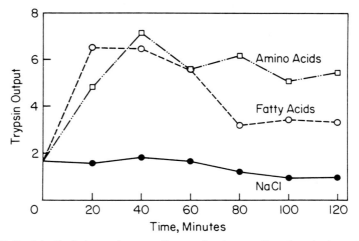

FIGURE 5–8.   Intestinal phase of pancreatic secretion in man. Trypsin output was increased by duodenal perfusion with amino acids and micellar fatty acids. The elevated trypsin levels produced by amino acid perfusion were equal to those attained by cholecystokinin infusion. (Modified from Go, V.L., Hofmann, A.F., and Summerskill, W.H.: Pancreozymin bioassay in man based on pancreatic enzyme secretion: Potency of specific amino acids and other digestive products. J. Clin. Invest., 49:1558, 1970.)

that the bicarbonate and volume response to intraluminal acid is significantly potentiated by simultaneous intraenteric placement of a potent stimulant of cholecystokinin release (i.e., phenylalanine). This potentiation is reduced by vagotomy, indicating that a cholinergic reflex also contributes to the overall response. The hormone potentiation effect on pancreatic bicarbonate and water secretion is assured by the ability of intraluminal acid to release small amounts of cholecystokinin along with secretin.

Cholecystokinin, a potent stimulant of pancreatic enzyme secretion, is released from the I cells of the intestinal mucosa by the products of fat and protein digestion (Fig. 5–8). Undigested lipids or proteins do not stimulate the release of cholecystokinin. The circulating levels of cholecystokinin are directly related to the concentration of the luminal stimulants and the length of the gut exposed to them. The most potent lipid stimulants are the long-chain fatty acids, their individual ability to release cholecystokinin being inversely related to the speed at which they are absorbed. Various peptides containing glycine and amino acids with aromatic residues (glycylphenylalanine, glycyltrypto-phan), as well as some essential amino acids (e.g., phenylalanine, methionine, valine) are also potent stimulants of cholecystokinin release. Carbohydrates do not affect cholecystokinin secretion. Since small amounts of secretin are also released by the products of lipid and protein digestion, secretin can potentiate the postprandial effects of cholecystokinin on pancreatic acinar cells.

Although it is clear that the hormones secretin and cholecystokinin are important determinants of the intestinal phase of pancreatic secretion, much less is known of the contribution of an enteropancreatic reflex. There are data which suggest that the enhanced pancreatic enzyme secretion induced by intraluminal perfusion with long-chain fatty acids or essential amino acids can be significantly reduced by vagotomy or atropine administration. Furthermore, the time of onset of the enhanced enzyme secretion is much shorter than the time required for the secreted hormones to reach the gland and elicit a response. Thus, the enteropancreatic reflex may serve to elicit a prompt pancreatic response to intraluminal nutrients; the subsequently released hormones serve to maintain the enhanced pancreatic secretion.

It is apparent that the intestinal phase of pancreatic secretion is complex, being the result of additive and potentiating effects of hormones (secretin and cholecystokinin) and neural activity (vago-vagal reflexes) on pancreatic secretory cells. Despite these multiple interactions, the enhanced pancreatic enzyme secretion produced by a meal peaks at levels about 70 per cent of the maximal rates of enzyme secretion attainable with exogenous hormonal stimulation. The inability of luminal stimulants to elicit a maximal response has been attibuted either to inadequate excitatory mechanisms or to the presence of inhibitory mechanisms. An increased rate of entrance of chyme into the duodenum does not increase pancreatic enzyme output to maximum rates, indicating that the intestine may not be sufficiently exciting the pancreas via neural and humoral mechanisms. Alternatively, there is evidence that intraluminal trypsin, hormones secreted postprandially by the ileal and colonic mucosa (e.g., pancreatone), and pancreatic hormones (somatostatin, pancreatic polypeptide, and glucagon) can inhibit pancreatic secretion (Table 5–2).

FUNCTIONS OF PANCREATIC JUICE

Bicarbonate

During a meal, the stomach can secrete as much as 20 to 40 mEq of hydrogen ions per hour. Despite the buffering capacity of ingested proteins and peptides, the pH of chyme is lowered to 2. Since the duodenal mucosa does not possess the protective barrier present in the stomach, the entrance of acidic chyme (containing pepsins) can result in ulcerations of the intestinal mucosa. Furthermore, the digestion of nutrients is impaired by an acidic chyme, since pancreatic enzymes require a pH between 6.0 to 8.0 for optimum activity. Indeed, lipase can be irreversibly inactivated when lumen pH falls below 4.0. Fortunately, the secretin-stimulated pancreas can secrete bicarbonate at a rate sufficient to neutralize all of the titratable acid delivered to the duodenum from the stomach. The bicarbonate ions (which enter the intestinal lumen from duodenal secretions and bile) also dissipate some of the acid entering the duodenum. However, the neutralizing capacity of the nonpancreatic secretions is minimal compared with that of pancreatic bicarbonate. Without the pancreas, the entire duodenum is acidified, whereas under normal conditions, most of the acid is dissipated at the level of the duodenal bulb.

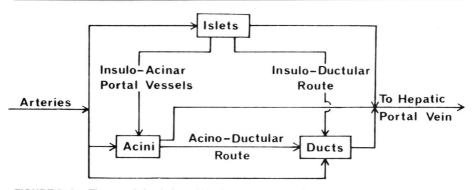

FIGURE 5–9.   The portal circulation within the pancreas. (From Ohtani, O., Kikuta, A., Ohtsuka, A., Taguchi, T., and Murakami, T.: Microvasculature as studied by the microvascular corrosion casting/scanning electron microscope method. I. Endocrine and digestive system. Arch. Histol. Jpn., *46*:1–42, 1983.)

Enzymes

Pancreatic juice contains a variety of digestive enzymes capable of hydrolyzing the major constituents of ingested food (Table 5–1). The pancreas normally secretes about ten times more enzyme than is required to hydrolyze all of the ingested nutrients to products that can be handled by the digestive (brush border and intracellular) enzymes and transport processes of the intestinal mucosa. Despite alternative sources of digestive enzymes (saliva and gastric juice), significant maldigestion and malabsorption occurs in the absence of pancreatic enzymes. Although patients can survive without pancreatic enzymes, health is impaired: body weight and muscle mass are reduced, and the patient is incapacitated by diarrhea associated with steatorrhea.

THE PANCREATIC CIRCULATION

The arterial supply of the pancreas is derived from the superior mesenteric artery (via the inferior pancreaticoduodenal artery) and the celiac artery (via the superior pancreaticoduodenal artery and pancreatic branches of the splenic artery). Within the gland, arterioles supply three distinct capillary plexuses: the acinar, ductular, and islet vascular beds (Fig. 5–9). The intrapancreatic circulation is also characterized by an extensive portal system. The acinar capillary plexus receives blood from vessels draining the islet plexus. The ductular plexus receives blood from vessels draining the acini and islets. All three vascular plexuses eventually drain into either the splenic vein or superior mesenteric vein; these, in turn, empty into the portal vein.

Functional Implications of a Portal Circulation

The intrapancreatic portal circulation illustrated in Figure 5–9 allows the hormones secreted by the endocrine portion of the pancreas (islets of Langerhans) to reach the exocrine portion of the gland (acinar and duct cells) in very high concentrations. The hormones released from islet cells are proteins of low molecular weight (insulin, 6000; glucagon, 3550; somatostatin, 1638; pancreatic polypeptide, 4250) that are small enough to filter across the fenestrated capillaries surrounding the ducts and acini in significant quantities. All of the pancreatic hormones are known to influence pancreatic exocrine secretion. Insulin enhances the synthesis and release of amylase and potentiates the secretory effects of cholecystokinin. Glucagon inhibits enzyme secretion, while somatostatin and pancreatic polypeptide inhibit bicarbonate and water secretion. In view of experimental findings, current opinion holds that the islets of Langerhan represent a "controlling center" for the exocrine function of the pancreas.

Role of the Microcirculation in Pancreatic Secretion

The pancreas is capable of secreting approximately 0.4 ml of juice per min per 100 grams of tissue during maximal stimulation induced by secretin. This rate of fluid secretion is approximately 30 times higher than the normal rate of capillary filtration in the pancreas. There is evidence that the Starling forces governing fluid exchange across pancreatic capillaries are altered during periods of enhanced secretion. After a meal, there is a doubling of pancreatic blood flow via mechanisms similar to those implicated in the salivary gland, i.e., increases in tissue metabolites, osmolality, or kinins (see Fig. 2–9). The arteriolar dilatation results in an increased capillary hydrostatic pressure which, in turn, provides the driving force for the movement of fluid from blood to ducts. Since, in some cases, pancreatic secretion can increase substantially without an accompanying increase in blood flow (and capillary pressure), the fluid for secretion can also be derived from the capillaries by changing the interstitial forces, i.e., increasing interstitial oncotic pressure and decreasing interstitial hydrostatic pressure. Such changes in the interstitial forces should result from the interstitial dehydration which occurs when the ductal epithelium transports water from the interstitial spaces into the duct lumen. During a meal, it is likely that both capillary and interstitial forces serve to support the ongoing pancreatic secretion.

PANCREATIC PAIN

Pain is a prominent feature of pancreatic disease. Pancreatic pain is felt in the upper abdomen, centrally, and in both the right and left subcostal regions. The pain frequently radiates to the back and relief is often obtained by sitting up and bending forward.

CLINICAL CORRELATIONS

The loss of exocrine and endocrine function that occurs in severe chronic pancreatitis produces a clinical picture which clearly illustrates the normal physiologic role of the pancreas. Chronic pancreatitis is often associated with alcoholism or biliary tract disease. This condition results in progressive loss, first of exocrine and subsequently of endocrine tissue of the gland, and the affected cells are replaced by fibrous tissue. In advanced cases, calcification of the parenchyma occurs, and this can be recognized in plain x-ray films of the abdomen.

Severe loss of exocrine function results in malabsorption and weight loss. The malabsorption involves proteins, long-chain triglycerides, fat-soluble vitamins, and trace elements, with the exception of iron. Protein malabsorption may be manifest as "starvation" edema. Malabsorption of fat results in steatorrhea, i.e., daily stool fat output of more than 5 grams when 100 grams of dietary fat is consumed daily. The stools are characteristically pale, bulky, and offensive. The action of colonic bacteria on unabsorbed lipids and proteins is responsible for the formation of malodorous compounds. Bacterial action on unabsorbed fats produces hydroxy-fatty acids similar to ricinoleic acid, the active principal of castor oil. These fatty acid derivatives cause water and electrolyte secretion by the colonic mucosa. In severe chronic pancreatitis, stool fat output may exceed 40 grams per day and this high output is due to the fact that triglyceride digestion by pancreatic lipase is a necessary prerequisite for fat absorption. However, only about 33 per cent of patients with chronic pancreatitis have steatorrhea as defined above. This is explained by the fact that the pancreas has a large functional reserve. When more than 90 per cent of exocrine function is lost, severe maldigestion and, consequently, malabsorption ensue.

As chronic pancreatitis progresses, endocrine tissue is also eventually lost with the development of frank diabetes mellitus; before reaching this stage, however, many patients will have already developed an abnormal glucose tolerance test.

The diagnosis of chronic pancreatitis is often established by intubation studies; a catheter is placed in the duodenal lumen and the pancreas is stimulated to secrete juice in response to a test meal or to intravenous administration of secretin and cholecystokinin. Measurements of bicarbonate and enzyme secretion are obtained from the aspirates. Frequently, an impaired output of bicarbonate in response to secretin is the earliest sign of pancreatic insufficiency.

Endoscopic cannulation of the pancreatic duct is used to demonstrate radiologically visible abnormalities of the duct system in chronic pancreatitis (irregularity, tortuosity, and focal dilatations). At the same time, samples of pancreatic juice can be obtained. A high level of lactoferrin in this pancreatic juice points to chronic pancreatitis. The reason for the elevated levels of lactoferrin in pancreatitis is unknown.

The replacement of exocrine function in patients with chronic pancreatitis can be achieved with oral preparations of freeze-dried animal pancreas extracts. These preparations should not contain free trypsin, since this enzyme can destroy other enzymes even in the stored dry state. Since the enzyme preparations are taken orally with meals, they have to run the gauntlet of gastric acid. Below a pH of 4, many pancreatic enzymes (e.g., lipase) are irreversibly inactivated. For this reason, it has become common to coadminister agents such as cimetidine to reduce gastric acid secretion and allow the pancreatic enzymes to survive until they reach the duodenal lumen.

REFERENCES

Berne, R.M., and Levy, M.N.: Physiology. St. Louis, C.V. Mosby Co., 1983.

Davenport, H.W.: Physiology of the Digestive Tract. Chicago, Year Book Medical Publishers, 1977.

Desnuelle, P., and Figarella, C.: Biochemistry. *In* Howat, H.T., and Sarles, H. (eds.): The Exocrine Pancreas. London, W.B. Saunders Co., 1979, pp. 86–125.

Garlick, F.S., and Jamieson, J.D.: Structure-function relationships of the pancreas. *In* Johnson, L.R. (ed.): Physiology of the Gastrointestinal Tract, Vol. 2. New York, Raven Press, 1981, pp. 773–794.

Harper, A.A., and Scratcherd, T.: Physiology. *In* Howat, H.T., and Sarles, H. (eds.): The Exocrine Pancreas. London, W.B. Saunders Co., 1979, pp. 50–85.

Henderson, J.R., Daniel, P.M., and Fraser, P.A.: The pancreas as a single organ: The influence of the endocrine upon the exocrine part of the gland. Gut, 22:158–167, 1981.

Johnson, L.R. (ed.): Gastrointestinal Physiology. St. Louis, C.V. Mosby Co., 1981.

Kern, R., and Blum, A.L. (eds.): The Gastroenterology Annual, Vol. 1. Amsterdam, Elsevier, 1983.

Kvietys, P.R., Patterson, W.G., and Granger, D.N.: Intrinsic and extrinsic regulation of the pancreatic microcirculation. *In* Courtice, F.C., Garlick, D.G., and Perry, M.A. (eds.): Progress in Microcirculation Research, Vol. 2. Sydney, University of South Wales, 1984.

Meyer, J.H.: Pancreatic physiology. *In* Sleisenger, M.H., and Fordtran, J.S. (eds.): Gastrointestinal Disease, 3rd ed. Philadelphia, W.B. Saunders Co., 1983, pp. 1426–1436.

Meyer, J.H.: Regulation of pancreatic exocrine secretion. *In* Johnson, L.R. (ed.): Physiology of the Gastrointestinal Tract, Vol. 2. New York, Raven Press, 1981, pp. 821–829.

Ohtani, O., Ohtsuka, A., and Murakami, T.: Microvascular organization of the pancreas. *In* Koo, A., Lam, S.K., and Smaje, L.H. (eds.): Microcirculation of the Alimentary Canal. Singapore, World Scientific, 1983, pp. 29–38.

Schulz, I.: Electrolyte and fluid secretion in the exocrine pancreas. *In* Johnson, L.R. (ed.): Physiology of the Gastrointestinal Tract, Vol. 2. New York, Raven Press, 1981, pp. 795–819.

Interposed between the digestive tract and other organ systems, the liver functions to store, metabolize, and distribute (via blood) the large amount of nutrients which are ingested in the form of food. The liver also interacts with the digestive system by secreting bile, a solution of detergent molecules called bile salts. Bile is concentrated and stored in the gallbladder during the interdigestive period. The presence of fat in intestinal chyme leads to gallbladder contraction and the delivery of bile into the gut lumen, an effect mediated by the hormone cholecystokinin. While present in the gut lumen, bile promotes the efficient digestion and absorption of lipids. The bile salts and other constituents of bile are absorbed in the small bowel and returned to the liver via the portal vein for resecretion into bile. In addition to its role in fat digestion, bile excretion provides a major route for the elimination of endogenous compounds (e.g., cholesterol and bilirubin), drugs, and environmental pollutants.

6

THE LIVER AND BILIARY TREE

ANATOMY OF THE BILIARY TREE

The biliary tree starts blindly with the bile canaliculi, which are small channels approximately 1 μm in diameter formed by the fusion of the plasma membranes of adjacent hepatocytes. The canaliculi have no epithelium, yet their walls are elongated by the formation of fingerlike microvilli, which greatly increase the area available for bile secretion. Bile canaliculi drain into the ducts of Herring (also known as preductules), which in turn connect to ductules and ducts. The biliary ductules and ducts are lined by small cuboidal epithelial cells which exhibit characteristic features of a secretory cell such as microvilli and micropinocytotic vesicles. Within the liver, the bile ducts merge and increase in diameter as they travel with branches of the hepatic artery and portal vein. The epithelium gradually changes from a cuboidal to a columnar type as the ducts increase in diameter.

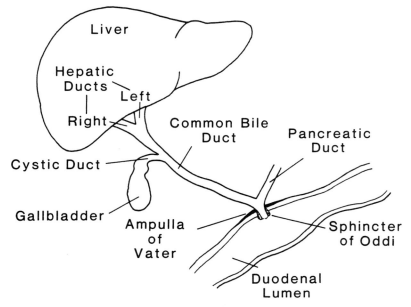

FIGURE 6–1. The biliary system.

The extrahepatic biliary system in man consists of the (1) hepatic bile ducts (right and left), (2) cystic duct, (3) common bile duct, and (4) gallbladder (Fig. 6–1). The two hepatic ducts join with the cystic duct from the gallbladder to form the common bile duct, which empties into the small intestine at the duodenal papilla (ampulla of Vater). At the entrance of the bile duct into the duodenum there is a thickening of the circular muscle of the duct which is called the sphincter of Oddi. The sphincter governs the diameter of the bile duct orifice in the ampulla and, thereby, controls the rate of bile flow into the gut lumen.

The gallbladder is a thin muscular organ that forms a blind appendage of the common bile duct. The inner wall of the gallbladder is lined by a single layer of tall, columnar epithelium and is characterized by folds analogous to intestinal villi. The human gallbladder is not a large organ; when full it can only accommodate 40 to 50 ml of fluid.

Hepatocyte Growth and Regeneration

The liver has an enormous capacity for regeneration after partial resection. Indeed, this model has been extensively used in experimental studies of cell division and growth. Mitotic figures in hepatocytes of normal liver are scarce, but in the regenerating liver every hepatocyte will divide in a period of 24 hours. The major trophic influences on the liver are insulin, glucagon, and epidermal growth factors. The importance of insulin and glucagon in main-

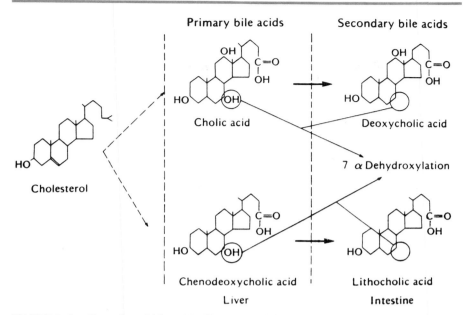

Primary bile acids   Secondary bile acids

Cholic acid   Deoxycholic acid

Cholesterol

7 α Dehydroxylation

Chenodeoxycholic acid   Lithocholic acid

Liver   Intestine

FIGURE 6–2. Formation of bile acids. The primary bile acids (cholic and chenodeoxycholic acids) are synthesized from cholesterol in the liver. Secondary bile acids (deoxycholic and lithocholic acids) are formed by dehydroxylation of primary bile acids by bacteria in the intestine. (From Williams, C.N. *In* Brooks, F.P. (ed.): Gastrointestinal Pathophysiology. New York, Oxford University Press, 1974, p. 160.)

taining normal liver structure is underscored by the hepatic atrophy that results from diversion of pancreatic venous blood from the liver.

COMPOSITION OF BILE

Hepatic Bile

Like most other exocrine secretions, bile is an aqueous solution of organic and inorganic compounds (see Table 6–1). The concentrations of electrolytes in hepatic bile resemble those in plasma, with the exception that bicarbonate concentration may be twice as high. It is the presence of organic compounds that distinguishes hepatic bile from plasma. Bile also contains small amounts of proteins, most of which are plasma proteins.

Bile acids in human hepatic bile can be divided into primary and secondary (Fig. 6–2). Primary bile acids are synthesized from cholesterol by hepatocytes. The conversion of cholesterol to bile acids primarily involves the addition of hydroxyl groups and a carboxyl group to the steroid nucleus, which increases the water solubility of bile acids relative to cholesterol. The major primary bile acids in man are cholic acid (a trihydroxycholanic acid) and chenodeoxycholic acid (a dihydroxycholanic acid).

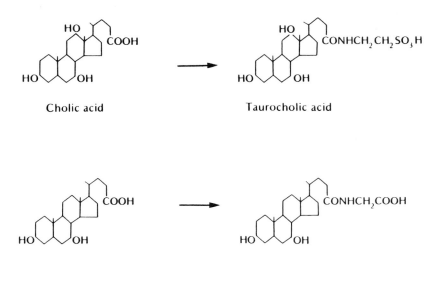

FIGURE 6–3. Conjugation of primary bile acids. Cholic acid is conjugated with taurine while chenodeoxycholic acid is conjugated with glycine.

Secondary bile acids are formed by dehydroxylation of primary bile acids by bacteria in the digestive tract. Bacterial metabolism of bile salts requires the presence of obligate anaerobes in concentrations above 10^4 per cu mm. Such conditions normally occur in the distal ileum, cecum, and colon. The secondary bile acids are absorbed in the distal bowel and returned to the liver via the portal vein where they are secreted into bile. The major secondary bile acids in man are deoxycholic acid and lithocholic acid. Cholic acid, chenodeoxycholic acid, and deoxycholic acid normally appear in a ratio of 4:4:2 in hepatic bile, while lithocholic acid is usually present only in small quantities (10 to 20 per cent of the deoxycholic acid concentration). The low concentration of lithocholic acid results from its insolubility and consequent poor absorption in the distal bowel.

Both primary and secondary bile acids are conjugated with either glycine or taurine in the liver (Fig. 6–3). The concentration of glycine conjugates is approximately two to three times higher than that of taurine conjugates in human bile, presumably due to the limited availability of taurine in the diet. Conjugated bile acids ionize more readily than free bile acids and therefore exist as salts of various cations, e.g., sodium taurocholate. Conjugated bile acids are more water soluble than unconjugated bile acids, with taurine conjugates exhibiting a greater solubility than glycine conjugates. When pH falls below 4.0, glycine-conjugated bile salts precipitate out of solution; however, the alkaline nature of biliary and pancreatic secretions prevents this from occurring

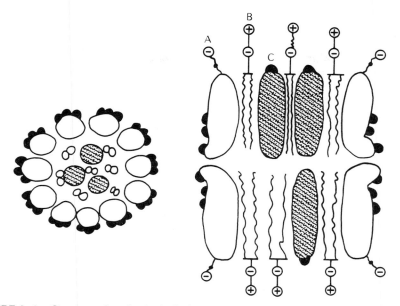

FIGURE 6–4. Structure of a mixed micelle in longitudinal (*right*) and cross section (*left*). The micelle consists of bile acids (A), lecithin (B), and cholesterol (C). The water-soluble aspect of the bile acids covers the sides of the micelle while cholesterol and the nonpolar portion of the phospholipid are solubilized in the hydrophobic interior of the micelle. (From Brooks, F.P.: Gastrointestinal Pathophysiology, 2nd ed. New York, Oxford University Press, 1978, p. 240.)

in the biliary tract and intestine, respectively. Conjugated bile salts are rarely present in the feces because bacteria in the distal ileum and colon deconjugate the bile salts.

Three-dimensional analyses of conjugated and unconjugated bile acid molecules reveal that the hydroxyl groups are all on the same side of the molecule while the water-insoluble portion of the molecule is on the opposite surface. This configuration imparts amphipathic properties to the bile acid; i.e., it has both hydrophilic and hydrophobic domains. Because of their amphipathic properties, bile acids tend to form molecular aggregates known as micelles when their concentration exceeds a critical level (called the critical micellar concentration). In micelles, the bile acid molecules are oriented so that the hydrophilic portion of the molecule faces the aqueous phase of the solution while the hydrophobic portion faces inward, away from the aqueous phase. Therefore, the interior of the micelle becomes a lipid-soluble environment where lipids such as cholesterol, which are very water-insoluble, can be maintained in a solution such as bile. In normal bile, bile acids, cholesterol, and phospholipids exist in the form of "mixed micelles" (Fig. 6–4). The concentration of bile acids in hepatic bile is normally well above the critical micellar concentration (2 to 5 mM), thereby ensuring an appropriate environment for solubilization of cholesterol and phospholipids.

Phospholipids and cholesterol comprise approximately 20 per cent and 4 per cent of the total solutes in hepatic bile, respectively. Lecithin accounts for 98 per cent of the phospholipids with the remainder consisting of sphingomyelin, cephalin, and lysolecithin. Both lecithin and cholesterol are essentially insoluble in water; however, they are solubilized in bile acid micelles. Cholesterol, a nonpolar molecule, dissolves in the center of the micelle while lecithin, which is amphipathic, partitions its fatty acyl chains into the center and leaves its polar head near the surface of the micelle. A "mixed micelle" of bile acids and lecithin has a greater capacity for solubilizing cholesterol than has a simple bile acid micelle. When the concentration of cholesterol in bile is greater than can be solubilized, crystals of cholesterol are formed. This crystallization of cholesterol plays an important role in the formation of cholesterol gallstones.

Bile pigments account for the golden yellow color of bile. Bilirubin, an end-product of hemoglobin degradation, is the principal pigment of bile. The bile pigments are essentially insoluble in water unless conjugated with another substance. Bilirubin is conjugated primarily with glucuronic acid (80 per cent) and, to a lesser extent (10 per cent), with sulfate by hepatocytes. Upon excretion into the bowel lumen, conjugated bilirubin is converted by bacterial action to highly soluble substances such as urobilinogen, which can be reabsorbed by the intestine or oxidized in the feces to stercobilin. The end-products of bile pigment degradation by bacteria such as stercobilin are responsible for the brown color of the stool.

A variety of other organic and inorganic compounds normally appear in bile in minute quantities. These compounds include lipids, steroid hormones (e.g., estrogens), and end-products of drug and hormone metabolism. Small amounts of heavy metals, such as lead and arsenic (and other environmental pollutants), also appear in bile, and the elimination of these substances by the biliary system may provide an important level of protection against their toxic effects.

Gallbladder Bile

Table 6–1 compares the composition of gallbladder bile to that of hepatic bile. There are several major differences in the bile compositions, all of which are related to the absorptive functions of the gallbladder. The concentrations of cations, bile acids, lecithin, bile pigments, and cholesterol are much higher in gallbladder bile than hepatic bile. This difference results primarily from the reduction in the volume of bile in the gallbladder caused by water absorption. The concentrations of Cl^- and HCO_3^- in gallbladder bile are significantly less than in hepatic bile. These differences are attributed to Cl^- and HCO_3^- absorption. Because of HCO_3^- absorption, the pH of gallbladder bile is lower than that of hepatic bile as well as plasma. Gallbladder bile remains isotonic with plasma despite the dramatic rise in electrolyte and bile acid concentrations. The fact that micelles have minimal osmotic activity, coupled to their ability

TABLE 6–1. Comparison of Hepatic and Gallbladder Bile Composition

Constituent	Hepatic Bile (mM)	Gallbladder Bile (mM)
Na$^+$	165	280
K$^+$	5	10
Ca^{++}	2.5	12
Cl$^-$	90	15
HCO$_3^-$	45	8
Bile acids	35	310
Lecithin	1	8
Bile pigments	0.8	3.2
Cholesterol	3	25
pH	8.2	6.5

to sequester counter-ions such as sodium, explains the maintenance of isotonicity even though there is a larger concentration of solutes in gallbladder bile.

MECHANISMS OF HEPATIC BILE FORMATION

The liver of adult man normally produces approximately 600 ml (range, 250 to 1100 ml) of bile per day, with an average rate of 0.42 ml/min. Roughly 75 per cent of hepatic bile is formed at the bile canaliculi while the remaining 25 per cent is secreted by the bile ducts. The canalicular component of bile formation can be divided into two fractions: a bile acid–dependent fraction, which accounts for 0.15 ml/min of the hepatic bile flow, and a bile acid–independent fraction, which accounts for 0.16 ml/min of total hepatic bile flow (Fig. 6–5).

Canalicular Bile Formation

BILE ACID–DEPENDENT SECRETION

Canalicular bile formation is generally regarded as an osmotic water flow in response to active solute transport (Fig. 6–6). Because of the excellent correlation between bile flow and bile acid secretion (Fig. 6–5), bile acids are considered to be one of the solutes generating bile flow. Bile acids are secreted against a concentration gradient; their biliary concentration is 100 to 1000 times higher than their plasma concentration. The secretion of bile acids into the canalicular lumen probably takes place through a carrier-mediated process. An osmotic gradient is established between the canalicular lumen and the hepatic interstitial space owing to the osmotic activity of the bile acids (or of their associated counter-ions) secreted into the canaliculus. The osmotic pressure gradient draws water through the hepatocyte and the intercellular spaces (tight junctions) and into the lumen, thereby leading to the formation of isotonic bile (see Fig. 1–13 for discussion of standing osmotic gradient theory).

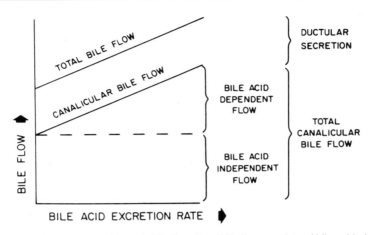

FIGURE 6–5.   Components of hepatic bile flow. Total bile flow consists of bile acid–dependent canalicular secretion, bile acid–independent canalicular secretion, and ductular secretion. Total canalicular bile flow represents the difference between total bile flow and ductular secretion. Bile acid–independent *canalicular* secretion is defined as the canalicular bile flow when bile acid excretion rate is zero. (From Scharschmidt, B.F. *In* Zakim, D., and Boyer, T. (eds.): Hepatology. Philadelphia, W.B. Saunders, 1982.)

The bile acids which are actively secreted into the canaliculi are derived either by *de novo* synthesis from cholesterol or by extraction from portal venous blood. The rate-limiting reaction in the conversion of cholesterol to primary bile acids is the hydroxylation step catalyzed by the enzyme 7-α hydroxylase. Feedback inhibition of bile acid synthesis by the concentration of bile acids in portal blood occurs at this step. Hepatocytes have a high extraction efficiency for bile acids; i.e., approximately 80 per cent of the bile acids in portal venous blood is taken up by the liver in a single pass. The uptake of bile acids by hepatocytes involves a carrier-mediated process which has a high transport maximum. Secretion of bile acids into the canaliculi, rather than hepatocellular uptake, is the rate-limiting step in overall transport of bile acids from blood to bile, inasmuch as the uptake velocity exceeds the secretory transport maximum by about sixfold.

The secretion of bilirubin, cholesterol, and phospholipid into bile also involves active transport processes. Bilirubin is actively extracted from blood by hepatocytes in proportion to its free (unconjugated) concentration in plasma. After bilirubin is conjugated within the hepatocyte, it is actively secreted into the canaliculus by an unknown mechanism. The mechanism(s) by which cholesterol and phospholipids are secreted into bile is also unknown; however, their rate(s) of secretion appears to be bile acid–dependent. The phospholipids secreted into bile are largely derived from synthetic mechanisms within the hepatocyte. Bile cholesterol, on the other hand, is derived from both the body pool of cholesterol and freshly synthesized cholesterol in the hepatocyte.

The ability of liver cells to secrete synthetic compounds which exhibit a

Plasma   Hepatocyte   Canaliculus

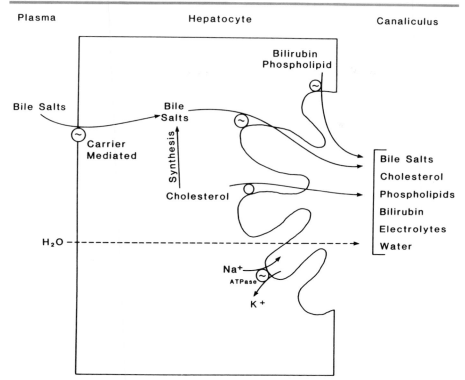

FIGURE 6–6. Mechanisms involved in bile acid–dependent and independent canalicular se-cretions. Active bile salt transport and the resultant osmotic water flow into the canaliculus are primarily responsible for the bile acid–dependent secretion. The bile acid–independent secretion results from active sodium transport into the canaliculus, a process energized by Na$^+$,K$^+$-ATPase.

transport maximum has been used as a crude test of liver function. Bromsul-phthalein (BSP), which is removed from the blood by hepatocytes and secreted into bile, is one such compound. The transport maximum for BSP, which is normally 8.0 mg per min, is reduced to nearly zero in patients with severe liver disease.

BILE ACID–INDEPENDENT SECRETION

There is considerable evidence suggesting that bile is also formed at the canaliculus by a mechanism which is independent of bile acid secretion. In-hibitors of the enzyme Na$^+$,K$^+$-ATPase completely block the bile acid–independent secretion, indicating that water movement coupled to active Na$^+$ secretion into the canaliculus is responsible for this fraction of bile for-

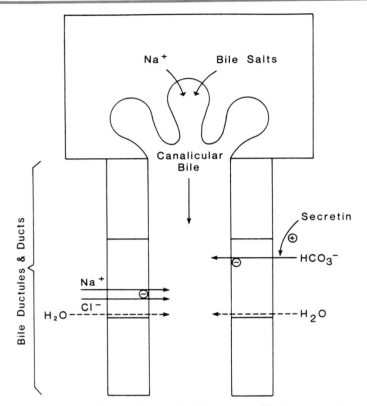

FIGURE 6–7. Mechanisms involved in ductular bile secretion. Bicarbonate, sodium, and chloride ions are actively secreted into the lumen of the bile ductules. Water moves passively across paracellular pathways owing to the osmotic gradient created by electrolyte transport.

mation (Fig. 6–6). The mechanism of coupling of the enzyme with solute and water transport has not been elucidated. There is evidence that a bicarbonate transport mechanism may also play a role in the elaboration of bile acid–independent secretion.

Ductal Component of Bile Flow

A number of studies on isolated perfused bile ducts indicate that a component of total bile flow results from electrolyte and water secretion by ductal epithelium (Fig. 6–7). The movement of water is coupled to active bicarbonate secretion and possibly an electroneutral sodium chloride pump. As a result of HCO_3^- secretion by the biliary epithelium, hepatic bile becomes alkaline. The hormone secretin is a potent stimulant of ductal HCO_3^- and water secretion. The quantitative significance of ductal secretion to total bile flow is highly species-dependent. Species which feed intermittently, such as man, have an important ductal contribution, whereas the ductal contribution is negligible in continuous eaters such as rodents.

The epithelium of the biliary ducts and ductules also has the capacity to absorb electrolytes and water. Although little is known concerning the mechanisms involved in water absorption by ductal epithelium, it appears that the common bile duct can take over a significant fraction of the gallbladder's concentrative capacity, e.g., following cholecystectomy in dogs. The relative importance of the secretory and absorptive functions of the ductal epithelium probably varies with the physiologic status of the individual.

FUNCTIONS OF THE GALLBLADDER

Once bile is formed at the canaliculi and ducts, it flows down the biliary tree and drains into either the gallbladder or the intestine. The force responsible for propelling bile down the biliary tree is the secretory pressure generated by the hepatocytes and ductal epithelia. Biliary secretion pressures as high as 10 to 20 mm Hg can be generated owing to active secretion of bile acids and electrolytes. During the interdigestive period, there is an increased resistance to bile flow in the common bile duct due to constriction of the sphincter of Oddi. The increased sphincteric tone, coupled with a relaxed gallbladder, allows the biliary secretion pressure to propel hepatic bile preferentially into the cystic duct and gallbladder. Storage of bile within the gallbladder during the interdigestive periods serves two important physiologic functions: (1) to concentrate bile, and (2) to deliver bile into the duodenum at the appropriate time after ingestion of food.

Water and Electrolyte Transport in the Gallbladder

As illustrated in Table 6–1 there are major differences in the composition of hepatic and gallbladder bile, which can be largely explained by water absorption in the gallbladder. In the fasted state, the human liver can secrete a volume of bile which is several times the fluid capacity of the gallbladder (20 to 50 ml). The ability of the gallbladder to concentrate bile some 5 to 20 times accounts, in part, for the discrepancy between the amount of bile secreted by the liver and the amount stored by the gallbladder. (Part of the discrepancy is explained by the fact that as much as 50 per cent of hepatic bile flow can drain into the duodenum in the interdigestive period.) Figure 6–8 illustrates the time required for conversion of hepatic bile into gallbladder bile. Within four hours up to 90 per cent of the water in hepatic bile is removed by the gallbladder.

Active sodium transport is primarily responsible for the ability of the gallbladder to concentrate bile. Sodium is transported, by a Na^+, K^+-ATPase activated pump located on the basolateral membrane of the epithelial cell, into the lateral intercellular space. Chloride and bicarbonate anions are also trans-

HEPATIC BILE   GALLBLADDER BILE

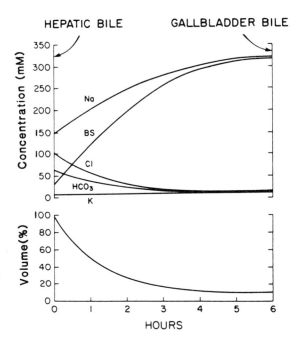

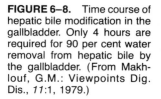

FIGURE 6–8. Time course of hepatic bile modification in the gallbladder. Only 4 hours are required for 90 per cent water removal from hepatic bile by the gallbladder. (From Makhlouf, G.M.: Viewpoints Dig. Dis., *11*:1, 1979.)

ported into the intercellular space to preserve electroneutrality; however, it is unclear whether the anion fluxes are due to an electrical potential difference created by an electrogenic Na^+ pump or whether a carrier couples the transport of the anions for each sodium ion pumped (an electroneutral pump). The high concentration of electrolytes (Na^+, Cl^-, and HCO_3^-) at the level of the lateral intercellular space creates a region of hypertonicity which provides a driving force for osmotic water flow from the gallbladder lumen to the mucosal interstitium. Because of the high water permeability of gallbladder epithelium, the degree of hypertonicity required to account for the high rate of water absorption is probably too small to measure experimentally.

The large volumes of water absorbed by the gallbladder epithelium have a "concentrating" effect on bile constituents which are either impermeable or only slightly permeable at the epithelial barrier. The resulting increase in bile concentrations of K^+, lecithin, conjugated bilirubin, and unconjugated bile salts creates a steeper gradient for passive diffusion of these "permeable" substances across gallbladder epithelium. This process allows for up to 20 per cent of bile lecithin and a smaller amount (< 5 per cent) of bile salts and bilirubin to be absorbed in the gallbladder. It is unclear whether the absorption of small quantities of organic bile constituents by the gallbladder is physiologically important.

An important modification of hepatic bile which takes place in the gallbladder is acidification. The pH of hepatic bile is approximately 8.2, and it is reduced to approximately 6.5 in the gallbladder. Two mechanisms have been proposed to explain the acidification of bile in the gallbladder: a hydrogen ion secretion mechanism and a HCO_3^- absorption mechanism. Both processes are likely to be involved; however, with current technology it is not possible to distinguish which of the two transport mechanisms is more important.

Motor Functions of the Gallbladder

In the interdigestive period, hepatic bile is diverted into the gallbladder where it is concentrated and stored until feeding. Shortly following a meal, the gallbladder contracts and the sphincter of Oddi relaxes. The resulting rise in biliary pressure and reduction in resistance to bile flow lead to the ejection of gallbladder bile into the duodenal lumen. Rhythmic contractions of the gallbladder musculature begin within 30 minutes after a meal and persist for up to 90 minutes. During the entire contraction period, the gallbladder discharges approximately 80 per cent of its contents into the duodenum.

The sphincter of Oddi exhibits an intrinsic electrical activity which is not synchronous with that of the longitudinal muscle of the duodenum. Bile flow from the common duct in humans is well correlated with the electrical activity of sphincteric muscle but not the duodenal muscle, indicating that the sphincter itself exerts primary control over the rate of bile excretion into the duodenum. Nonetheless, the contractile activity of the duodenum does influence bile flow. When the sphincter of Oddi is open, bile enters the bowel in spurts between periods of duodenal relaxation and contraction.

Ejection of bile into the duodenal lumen will occur during gallbladder contraction even in the absence of direct hormonal (CCK) relaxation of the sphincter of Oddi. This occurs as a result of the tendency for the sphincter to yield when the pressure in the common bile duct exceeds approximately 10 mm Hg. Contractions of the gallbladder can generate transient pressures exceeding 20 mm Hg in the biliary tree. Therefore, when the sphincter yields to such high pressures, bile spurts into the duodenal lumen. While this mechanism serves to ensure bile secretion and prevents marked elevations in biliary pressure during gallbladder contraction, it cannot generate the high rates of bile flow which are associated with a relaxed sphincter of Oddi.

THE ENTEROHEPATIC CIRCULATION

Fate of Bile Salts in the Intestine

When a meal is ingested, the gallbladder contracts and bile salts are secreted into the duodenal lumen. The concentration of bile salts in the duodenum during the early stage of gastric emptying is approximately half that of gallbladder bile. However, after gastric emptying, the luminal bile salt concentration is further reduced to approximately 10 mM owing to dilution with chyme. Even with the tenfold dilution of gallbladder bile, the concentration of bile salts in the intestinal lumen always remains above the critical micellar concentration. Pancreatic lipolysis of lecithin and triglycerides changes the composition of mixed micelles in the duodenal lumen. Here the mixed micelles are maximally enlarged with the products of lipid digestion, and larger spherical aggregates composed of the same lipids (called liposomes) are also formed.

An important function of the intestinal micelle is to solubilize the nonpolar products of luminal fat digestion within the polar environment of the gut lumen. The micelle facilitates the passive entry of the products of lipid digestion into the intestinal epithelial cell. Once the lipids move by simple diffusion across the brush border membrane, the bile salts remain within the bowel lumen where they are driven toward the ileum by intestinal motility.

Bile salts are absorbed in the small intestine by both passive diffusion and active transport. Passive diffusion of bile salts occurs along the entire length of the small intestine and colon. Estimates based on studies in primates and man suggest that as much as 50 per cent of the bile salts in the intestines are absorbed passively. Both conjugated and unconjugated bile salts undergo passive absorption. Glycine conjugates are more readily absorbed by simple diffusion than are taurine conjugates. Deconjugation and dehydroxylation of bile acids by bacteria in the distal ileum and colon enhance their lipid solubility and facilitate passive absorption. Deconjugation increases passive bile salt absorption ninefold while dehydroxylation increases it fourfold. The rate of deconjugation of glycine conjugates is over twice that of taurine conjugates.

Active absorption of bile salts occurs exclusively in the distal ileum. Like the absorption of most water-soluble substances, active bile salt transport is dependent upon the presence of sodium ions. A reciprocal relationship exists between active and passive transport rates of specific bile salts. The most polar bile salts (e.g., taurine conjugates), which are poorly absorbed by passive diffusion, have the highest active transport rates in the ileum. The active transport process for bile salts exhibits saturation kinetics, and there is competition among bile salts at the receptor (transport) sites.

Between 7 and 20 per cent of the total bile salt pool, i.e., the total amount of bile salts in the body at any given moment (approximately 3 grams), escapes absorption in the small and large bowel and is excreted in the feces. The fecal bile acids in health consist of deoxycholate and lithocholic acids (70 to 80 per cent) and unmetabolized primary bile salts, cholic and chenodeoxycholic acids (7 to 8 per cent). The daily fecal loss of these bile salts is equal to their rates of hepatic synthesis, thereby maintaining a constant total bile salt pool.

The rate of spillage of certain bile salts into the colon appears to play an important role in governing daily fecal water loss. The two major dihydroxy bile acids of human bile, deoxycholic acid and chenodeoxycholic acid, modulate this process. An increased luminal concentration (above 3 mM) of either of these bile acids in the colon causes diarrhea, while decreased concentrations are associated with constipation. While the physiologic significance of the cathartic properties of bile acids remains to be determined, it is rather clear that this process accounts for a major portion of the enhanced fecal water loss in patients with a surgically resected ileum.

Transport of Absorbed Bile Salts to Liver and Resecretion into Bile

Once bile acids are absorbed in the small intestine, they enter the blood circulation, i.e., the portal vein. In blood, bile acids are tightly bound to albumin (50 to 75 per cent) and specific lipoproteins (20 to 50 per cent). Free bile acids are more tightly bound to plasma proteins than are conjugated salts. In the fasted state, the bile salt concentration in portal venous blood is approximately 20 μM. After a meal, the portal venous blood concentration increases by two to seven times the fasting level.

The bile acids absorbed from the intestine are transported by the portal vein to the liver, where the hepatocytes are extremely efficient at clearing portal venous blood of bile acids. It is estimated that 80 per cent of the bile salts in the portal vein are extracted in a single pass through the liver. Hepatocellular uptake of bile acids is a carrier-mediated process in which the extent of uptake is directly related to the polarity of the bile acid. Once the bile acids enter the hepatocyte, the deconjugated bile acids are reconjugated and a portion of the secondary bile acids are rehydroxylated. Then the bile salts are resecreted into bile, along with newly synthesized bile acids, by the active transport process described earlier in this chapter.

The flow of bile salts from liver to intestine and back to the liver again is known as the *enterohepatic circulation* (Fig. 6–9). The major physiologic significance of the enterohepatic circulation is that the recycling and reuse of bile salts allows for efficient lipolysis and fat absorption with a limited total body pool of bile salts. An amount of bile salts twice the total body pool is required for efficient lipolysis of an average meal, while five times the total body pool is required following a meal with a very high fat content. Thus, the total amount of body bile salts must be cycled two to five times through the enterohepatic circulation following a meal. The rhythm of the enterohepatic circulation, its acceleration during eating and deceleration during fasting, is determined by the pattern of dietary intake. Most individuals eat three meals a day and sleep at night. Accordingly, the total body bile salt pool of man undergoes 4 to 12 cycles per day in the enterohepatic circulation.

A number of other substances which are secreted into bile also undergo recycling in the enterohepatic circulation. Endogenous substances which are recycled include fat-soluble vitamins. Indomethacin, cardiac glycosides, antibiotics, and phenolsulfonphthalein are examples of exogenous compounds which undergo recycling. Some substances, such as lithocholic acid and cholesterol, are poorly recycled in the enterohepatic circulation, thereby facilitating the elimination of these potentially deleterious compounds.

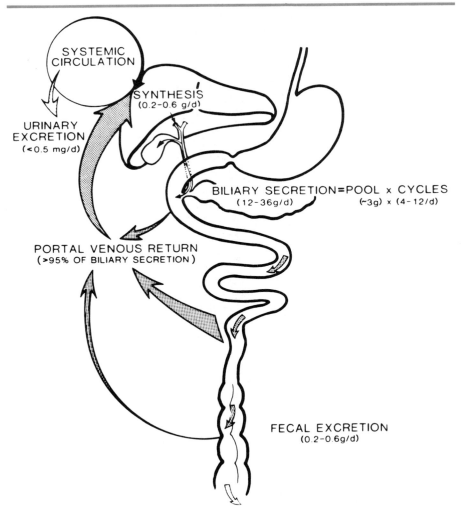

FIGURE 6–9. The enterohepatic circulation of bile salts in healthy man with typical kinetic values. (From Carey, M.C. *In* Arias, I., and Popper, H. (eds.): The Liver: Pathology and Pathobiology. New York, Raven Press, 1982, p. 433.)

REGULATION OF BILE FORMATION AND SECRETION

Bile Salt Concentration in Portal Blood

The major physiologic determinant of the rates of bile acid secretion and synthesis is the amount of bile acids in portal venous blood. As previously discussed, the concentration of bile acids in the hepatocyte exerts negative feedback control over the rate-limiting enzyme in bile acid synthesis (7 α-hydroxylase), and it is the primary regulator of the bile acid-dependent fraction of bile formation. The increased amount of bile acids in portal venous blood after a meal stimulates the secretion of bile acids (and bile flow) by the hepatocytes but inhibits the synthesis of bile acids. Conversely, interruption of the enterohepatic circulation (following ileal resection or ingestion of bile acid–binding agents such as cholestyramine) leads to a reduction in bile acid secretion (due to inadequate absorption) and a five- to tenfold increase in bile acid synthesis. A similar relationship beween synthesis and secretion is observed long after a meal, i.e., bile acid synthesis is maximal yet their rate of secretion is low, while the gallbladder fills slowly with bile.

Gastrointestinal Hormones

SECRETIN

Secretin is released from the duodenal mucosa in response to acidic chyme and subsequently exerts some influence over the transport functions of the bile ducts/ductules and gallbladder. Secretin stimulates the formation of an HCO_3^--rich and usually hypertonic fluid by the biliary ducts and ductules. The effects of secretin on biliary epithelium are believed to be mediated by cyclic AMP. The bile flow response to secretin is independent of the status of the enterohepatic circulation (bile acid concentration in portal venous blood). The responsiveness of the ductal system to secretin is species-dependent, with intermittent feeders (dog, man) being more responsive than continuous eaters (rat, rabbit). Bile flow increases threefold and bicarbonate output fourfold when secretin is administered to humans. The ductal responses to secretin are not mediated by vagal stimuli, since cholinergic blockade does not abolish the response to endogenous or exogenous secretin. Secretin also inhibits water and electrolyte reabsorption by the gallbladder. The lack of HCO_3^- reabsorption in the gallbladder, coupled with enhanced bicarbonate output by the ductal epithelium, may expedite the neutralization of acidic chyme in the duodenum. Finally, secretin causes gallbladder smooth muscle to contract; however, supraphysiologic concentrations are usually required to produce this effect.

CHOLECYSTOKININ

Cholecystokinin is released from the duodenal mucosa in response to the products of lipid digestion. It is the primary stimulus for gallbladder contraction and relaxation of the sphincter of Oddi following a meal. The hormone appears to act directly on both the smooth muscle of the gallbladder and the sphincter of Oddi. The smooth muscle of these structures is highly and specifically sensitive to cholecystokinin, compared to visceral smooth muscle in other regions of the G.I. tract. Isolated common bile ducts from human subjects also contract when exposed to cholecystokinin, suggesting that enhanced peristaltic contractions of the duct could further enhance bile flow in the postprandial state.

Although cholecystokinin has no effect on water and electrolyte transport in the gallbladder, it appears to stimulate bile flow in some species (dog). The mechanism of CCK-induced choleresis and its physiologic relevance remain uncertain.

OTHER HORMONES

Other hormones can also influence the rate of bile formation and secretion. Both gastrin and histamine stimulate bile flow by a direct action on the liver and indirectly by stimulating acid secretion by the stomach, which in turn releases secretin from the duodenal mucosa. Both substances induce a secretin-like increase in volume and bicarbonate secretion, yet neither causes gallbladder contraction. Glucagon, which is structurally similar to secretin, enhances bile formation yet, unlike secretin, does not increase bicarbonate concentration. Some steroid hormones, particularly estrogens and 19-alkylated androgens, inhibit bile formation by suppressing both bile acid–dependent and independent secretions. A reduction of bile formation is a well-known side effect of the therapeutic use of estrogen in human disease. The significant depression of bile acid secretion during pregnancy may be explained by high estrogen levels. Hydrocortisone, thyroxine, insulin, vasopressin, and prostaglandins also induce choleresis when administered in pharmacologic doses. Finally, recent studies suggest that motilin, which is released from the mucosa of the small bowel, may play an important role in modulating gallbladder contraction during the intestinal phase of digestion.

Nervous Influences

There are both vagal (parasympathetic) and sympathetic fibers supplying the biliary system. Vagal fibers travel in the hepatic branch of the anterior (right) vagal trunk and terminate on bile ducts as well as the myenteric plexus located in the submucosal and subserosal layers of the gallbladder. Cholinergic innervation of hepatic parenchymal cells is sparse. Sympathetic innervation of the biliary system is derived from the celiac plexus. Both efferent and afferent fibers are present. Sympathetic neurons supply the smooth muscle and myenteric plexus of the gallbladder and the bile ducts. Adrenergic innervation of hepatocytes is sparse; however, the intrahepatic blood vessels (portal venules, hepatic arterioles, and sinusoids) are richly innervated.

PARASYMPATHETICS

There is considerable evidence indicating that parasympathetic nerve activity influences the rate of both bile formation and gallbladder emptying. Acetylcholine administration and vagal stimulation both produce an increase in bile flow, which can be blocked by atropine. The increase in bile secretion observed after a meal is attenuated following bilateral vagotomy, suggesting that enhanced parasympathetic nerve activity accounts for a proportion of the secretory response to feeding. Cholinergic fibers from the vagi also appear to mediate the gallbladder contraction and sphincter of Oddi relaxation which occur during the cephalic and gastric phases of digestion. Acetylcholine administration and electrical stimulation of the parasympathetic nerves to the biliary tract produce both gallbladder contraction and relaxation of the sphincter of Oddi. Vagal stimulation also increases the maximal gallbladder contractile response to cholecystokinin, indicating an interaction between nervous and humoral mechanisms.

SYMPATHETICS

Intravenously administered catecholamines (e.g., norepinephrine) and stimulation of sympathetic nerves both cause a reduction in bile formation. However, it is unclear whether the effects of adrenergic stimulation on bile flow result from a direct influence on the biliary system, from indirect effects mediated by G.I. hormone release, or from alterations in blood flow. Sympathetic nerve stimulation causes relaxation of the gallbladder, yet the response of the sphincter of Oddi is variable. A physiologic role for sympathetic nerve activity in the regulation of biliary function appears unlikely.

Table 6–2 summarizes major aspects of control of the biliary system during the various phases of digestion.

THE HEPATIC CIRCULATION

Blood flow to the liver is derived from two sources, the portal vein and the hepatic artery. Within the liver, these vessels give rise to numerous smaller vessels called terminal portal venules and hepatic arterioles (Fig. 6–10). These terminal blood vessels supply a small mass of parenchyma called the liver acinus. The terminal portal venule and hepatic arteriole course along with a bile ductule (collectively called the portal axis) and enter the acinus at its center. The hepatic arterioles empty either (1) directly into the sinusoidal capillaries that lie between rows of hepatocytes or (2) into the peribiliary capillaries (supplying the bile ducts), which subsequently drain into the sinusoids. Since the portal venules also drain directly into the sinusoids, the hepatocytes are perfused with a mixture of venous and arterial blood. The sinusoids radiate toward the periphery of the acinus, where they drain into the larger central veins and ultimately into the hepatic veins and inferior vena cava.

The liver acinus can be subdivided into three circulatory zones which surround the portal axis as layers. Zone 1 encompasses the hepatocytes situated close to the portal axis and the origin of the sinusoid; hence, they are bathed by blood rich in nutrients and oxygen. The cells in Zone 3 are situated at the

TABLE 6–2.   Major Factors Affecting Gallbladder Emptying and Bile Synthesis and Secretion

Phase of Digestion	Stimulus	Mediating Factor	Response
Cephalic	Taste and smell of food; food in mouth and pharynx	Impulses in branches of vagus nerve (acetylcholine)	Increased rate of gallbladder emptying
Gastric	Gastric distention Nutrients	Impulses in branches of vagus nerve (acetylcholine), Gastrin	Increased rate of gallbladder emptying; increased rate of bile acid secretion
Intestinal	Fat digestion products in duodenum	Cholecystokinin	Increased rate of gallbladder emptying; increased rate of bile acid secretion
	Acid in duodenum	Secretin	Increased rate of secretion of electrolytes (HCO_3^-) and water by bile ducts; decreased rate of water and electrolyte absorption in gallbladder
	Absorption of bile acids in the distal part of ileum	High concentration of bile acids in portal blood	Stimulation of bile acid secretion; inhibition of bile acid synthesis
Interdigestive period	Low rate of release of bile into duodenum	Low concentration of bile acids in portal blood	Stimulation of bile acid synthesis; inhibition of bile acid secretion

periphery of the acinus, near the central vein. Hepatocytes in Zone 3 receive blood that has already exchanged nutrients and oxygen with cells in Zones 1 and 2 (the arbitrary intermediate zone). As a result of this microvascular organization, the metabolic requirements and transport functions of hepatocytes vary along the length of the sinusoid. Hepatocytes in Zone 1 are exposed to the highest blood oxygen tension and bile acid concentration. Therefore, these cells are most active for both oxidative metabolism and the uptake of bile acids. Conversely, the cells in Zone 3 are more geared for anaerobic metabolism, and the rate of bile acid uptake is low. It is also recognized that Zone 3 cells are most sensitive to damage due to ischemia, nutritional deficiency, and toxic substances (e.g., acetaminophen, carbon tetrachloride).

Under normal resting conditions in man, total hepatic blood flow accounts for approximately 25 per cent of cardiac output, i.e., 1250 to 1500 ml/min. The portal vein supplies the liver with 70 to 75 per cent of its blood; the hepatic artery provides the remaining 25 to 30 per cent. Because of the higher oxygen content in hepatic arterial blood, the hepatic artery and portal vein contribute an equal amount of oxygen to the liver in the fasting state. Hepatic blood flow increases following a meal, largely owing to an increased flow in the portal vein. The enterohepatic circulation of bile salts seems to influence liver blood

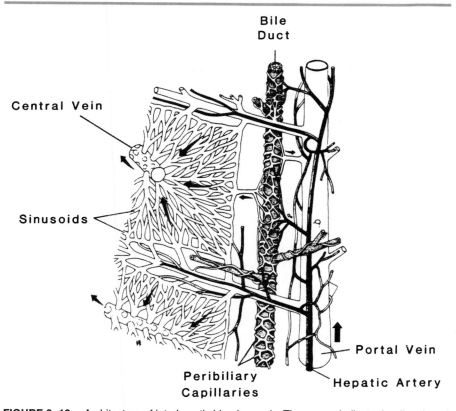

Bile Duct

Central Vein

Sinusoids

Portal Vein

Peribiliary Capillaries

Hepatic Artery

FIGURE 6–10. Architecture of intrahepatic blood vessels. The arrows indicate the direction of blood flow. (From Ohtani, O., Kikuta, A., Ohtsuka, A., Taguchi, T., and Murakami, T.: Microvasculature as studied by the microvascular corrosion casting/scanning electron microscope method. I. Endocrine and digestive system. Arch. Histol. Jpn., *46*:1–42, 1983.)

flow, inasmuch as an increased bile salt concentration in the portal vein causes hepatic arterial blood flow to rise.

The liver is probably the most important blood reservoir in man. The liver contains 25 to 30 ml of blood per 100 grams of tissue mass, accounting for 10 to 15 per cent of the total blood volume. Hepatic blood volume can expand to as much as 60 ml/100 grams of liver with cardiac failure. The capacitance function of the liver also plays an important role during hemorrhage. After a moderate blood loss with a drop in arterial pressure to 50 mm Hg, the liver expels enough blood to compensate for 25 per cent of the hemorrhage.

LIVER AND BILIARY PAIN

Pain arises from the liver only as a result of stretching the liver capsule and is experienced in a diffuse area over the right hypochondrium. Distention of either the common bile duct or the gallbladder results in pain experienced in the midepigastrium or the right subcostal region. Occasionally, pain from the biliary tract is experienced in the area below the scapula.

CLINICAL CORRELATIONS

Gallstones, which afflict about 20 million Americans (with a million new cases per year), represent a major medical and surgical problem. Gallstones result from the precipitation of insoluble material in bile. Cholesterol accounts for 80 per cent of gallstone material and bile pigment (calcium bilirubinate) for the remainder. Stones with varying mixtures of these two compounds are common. From a physiologic standpoint, the two aspects of this condition which are of chief interest are the pathogenesis or etiology and the medical management.

Pigment stones result from deconjugation of water-soluble bilirubin di-glucuronide by β-glucuronidase; insoluble bilirubin precipitates as its calcium salt. Beta-glucuronidase, present in bile, is normally inhibited by glucaric acid, also a bile constituent, and the precipitation of calcium bilirubinate may result from an imbalance between the enzyme and its inhibitor. This balance can be upset by additional β-glucuronidase derived from bacteria in an infected biliary tract. A large load of bilirubin resulting from hemolysis and excreted in the bile predisposes to the formation of pigment stones.

Despite the fact that it contains considerable amounts of cholesterol, which is essentially insoluble in water, normal bile is quite translucent. Cholesterol is held in solution in mixed phospholipid/bile salt micelles. This tripartite balance is quite precarious; a rise in the proportion of cholesterol to bile salts/phospholipids results in stone-forming (lithogenic) bile, when the capacity of the system to hold cholesterol in solution is exceeded. As crystals of cholesterol settle out from solution, stone formation begins. Clearly, either excessive cholesterol secretion or reduced output of bile salts/phospholipids can be responsible for this situation.

Women are about three times more likely than men to develop gallstones, and the incidence of the disease rises with increasing age in both sexes. Genetic factors seem to predispose to gallstones, as does obesity. Drugs which increase the biliary output of cholesterol, e.g., estrogens, the contraceptive pill, and the hypolipidemic drug clofibrate can cause gallstones. High carbohydrate diets also appear to favor the formation of gallstones. When the pool of bile salts and the concentration of bile salts in bile fall, as occurs when disease or resection of a substantial part of the distal ileum interferes with active bile salt reabsorption, gallstones form as a result of the reduced solubilizing capacity of bile for cholesterol. A good example of this is the occurrence of multiple gallstones in an otherwise healthy 16-year-old boy who, eight years previously, had undergone resection of a large segment of terminal ileum following a road accident (gallstones are ordinarily rather unusual in this sex and age group). Similarly,

Crohn's ileitis, a chronic inflammation of the terminal ileum where bile salts are actively absorbed, is a common predisposing situation for gallstone formation.

Traditionally, surgery (excision of the gallbladder and removal of stones from the biliary tree) has been the usual treatment for gallstones. However, in the past decade, there has been great interest in methods for manipulating the concentration of cholesterol relative to bile salts in bile and converting lithogenic to nonlithogenic bile, allowing dissolution of gallstones. This can be achieved by feeding chenodeoxycholic acid; the hepatic synthesis and secretion of cholesterol in bile falls. Weight reduction and limitation of carbohydrate intake may be useful adjuncts to this form of therapy, since these measures will also tend to favor the formation of nonlithogenic bile. The treatment tends to cause diarrhea when high doses of chenodeoxycholic acid are fed; this is due to the effect of bile salts on water and electrolyte transport by colonic mucosa.

REFERENCES

Berne, R.M., and Levy, M.N.: Physiology. St. Louis, C.V. Mosby Co., 1983.

Brooks, F.P.: Anatomy and physiology of the gallbladder and bile ducts. In Bockus, H.L. (ed.): Gastroenterology, 2nd ed., Vol. 3. Philadelphia, W.B. Saunders Co., 1976.

Carey, M.C.: The enterohepatic circulation. In Arias, I.M. (ed.): The Liver: Biology and Pathobiology. New York, Raven Press, 1982.

Davenport, H.W.: Physiology of the Digestive Tract. Chicago, Year Book Medical Publishers, 1977.

Erlinger, S.: Bile flow. In Arias, I.M. (ed.): The Liver: Biology and Pathobiology. New York, Raven Press, 1982.

Guyton, A.C.: Textbook of Medical Physiology, 6th ed. Philadelphia, W.B. Saunders Co., 1981.

Javitt, N.B. (ed.): Liver and Biliary Tract Physiology. International Review of Physiology, vol. 21. Baltimore, University Park Press, 1980.

Johnson, L.R. (ed.): Gastrointestinal Physiology. St. Louis, C.V. Mosby Co., 1981.

Scharschmidt, B.F.: Bile formation and gallbladder and bile duct function. In Sleisenger, M.H., and Fordtran, J.S. (eds.): Gastrointestinal Disease, 3rd ed. Philadelphia, W.B. Saunders Co., 1983.

Sernka, T.J., and Jacobson, E.D.: Gastrointestinal Physiology. The Essentials. Baltimore, Williams and Wilkins, 1983.

The small intestine is a tubular structure extending from the stomach to the colon. Its functions include mixing and propulsion of lumen contents, digestion and absorption of nutrients, secretion of hormones, and participation in the immune response. The first three of these functions play important roles in the overall process of assimilation of ingested food. The chyme entering the small intestine is thoroughly mixed with pancreatic and biliary secretions by contractions of the muscularis externa. The coordinated activity of the smooth muscle coat assures that chyme is gradually moved analward. Specialized endocrine cells in the mucosa secrete various hormones that regulate the amount and composition of digestive secretions delivered to the small intestine. The absorption of electrolytes, nutrients, and water is facilitated by the large surface area of the mucosa. Every 24 hours approximately 8 liters of water, partially hydrolyzed nutrients, and various secretions enter the small intestine, where most of it is absorbed.

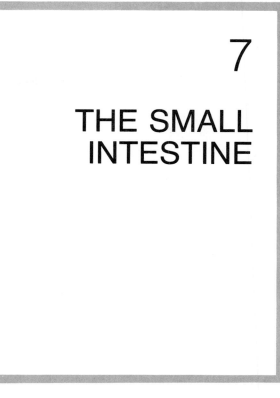

7

THE SMALL
INTESTINE

ANATOMY

The small intestine is about 6 to 7 meters in length when relaxed (post-mortem) and can be as short as 3 meters if tension is present (in vivo). Its diameter is about 4 centimeters but varies along the length of the gut, being larger in caliber in the proximal segments. The small bowel is often arbitrarily divided into three parts—the duodenum (the first 20 to 30 cm), jejunum (the second 2.5 meters), and the ileum (the final 3.5 meters). This division is somewhat imprecise, based at times on slight anatomic differences (presence of Brunner's glands in the duodenum) or functional differences (active transport of bile salts in the terminal ileum). The differences between these regions are not as obvious as are the similarities. At every level of the gut, the wall can be clearly partitioned into four basic layers: serosa, muscularis externa, submucosa, and mucosa (Fig. 7–1).

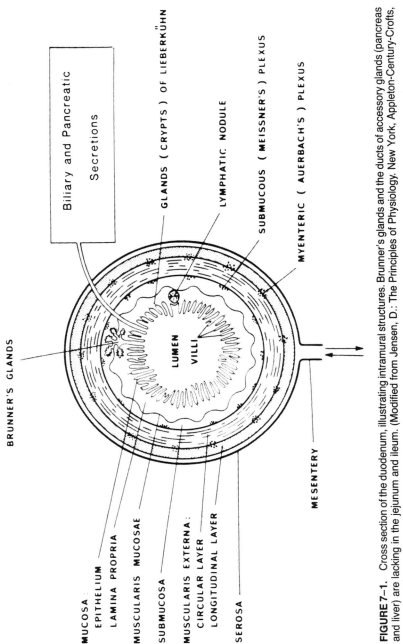

FIGURE 7–1.   Cross section of the duodenum, illustrating intramural structures. Brunner's glands and the ducts of accessory glands (pancreas and liver) are lacking in the jejunum and ileum. (Modified from Jensen, D.: The Principles of Physiology. New York, Appleton-Century-Crofts, 1976, p. 818.)

THE SMALL INTESTINE 143

Serosa

The outermost layer, the serosa, consists of simple squamous epithelium (mesothelium) which rests on connective tissue. The serosal lining is continuous with the abdominal peritoneum.

Muscularis Externa

The muscularis externa is composed of two well-defined layers of smooth muscle: a thinner outer layer which surrounds a thicker inner layer. Although all of the smooth muscle cells are spindle-shaped (200 μm long and 6 μm wide), their orientation differs in the two layers of smooth muscle. In the outer layer, the long axes of the cells are oriented in the longitudinal direction, while in the inner layer the long axes of the cells are oriented in a circular direction. Within each layer the smooth muscle cells are densely packed (180,000 cells per cu mm). The cells are separated mainly by small spaces (10 nm) which are occupied by collagen fibers and by a few larger spaces containing nerves, capillaries, interstitial cells, and connective tissue. In many cases, especially in the circular muscle layer, the plasma membranes of adjacent smooth muscle cells appear fused at various points, forming nexi. These nexi, occupying 6 per cent of the cell surface, allow for electrical coupling among the cells and muscle bundles. The presence of these nexi is particularly important, since bundles of smooth muscle cells (containing 200 to 400 cells), not individual cells, represent the smallest electrically excitable unit of visceral smooth muscle.

The longitudinal and circular muscle layers are separated by a connective tissue septum which varies greatly in thickness and contains the myenteric (Auerbach's) plexus and parasympathetic ganglion cells. The contractile and electrical activities of these two layers are coupled by means of connective tissue bridges and the myenteric plexus, respectively. Another plexus of nerve fibers (Meissner's plexus) is located in the submucosa adjacent to the circular smooth muscle layer. The Meissner's plexus may also play a role in coordinating the activity of the longitudinal and circular muscle layers.

Submucosa

The submucosa is a layer of loose connective tissue lying between the circular muscle layer and the muscularis mucosae. Contained in this layer are the larger blood vessels and lymphatics, as well as the ganglion cells and nerve fibers of Meissner's plexus. In the upper duodenum, the submucosa also contains elaborately branched acinar glands, the Brunner's glands. The serous and mucous cells of these glands elaborate a bicarbonate- and glycoprotein-rich secretion which is delivered to the duodenal lumen via short ducts passing through the mucosal layer. The alkaline nature of this secretion aids in neutralizing the acidic chyme entering the upper duodenum from the stomach. In lower portions of the duodenum and the remainder of the small intestine, the submucosal layer is largely devoid of glands.

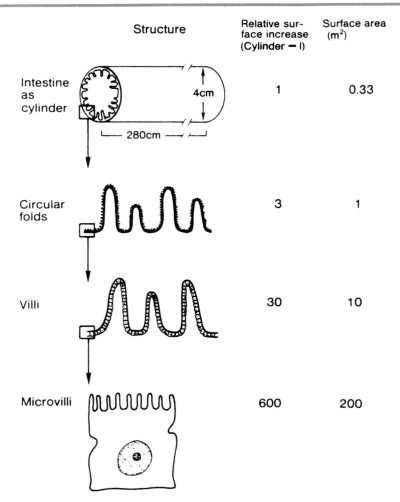

Structure	Relative sur-face increase (Cylinder – I)	Surface area (m²)
Intestine as cylinder	1	0.33
Circular folds	3	1
Villi	30	10
Microvilli	600	200

FIGURE 7–2.   Amplification of the mucosal surface area by specialized features of the mucosa. (From Schmidt, R.F., and Threws, G.: Human Physiology. Berlin, Springer-Verlag, 1983, p. 602.)

Mucosa

The mucosal layer, comprising the luminal surface of the small intestine, is designed to provide a large surface area for contact with lumen contents. Three anatomic modifications amplify the mucosal surface above that predicted for a simple cylinder (Fig. 7–2). Spiral or circular concentric folds called plicae circulares (or valvulae conniventes) contribute to this amplification. They are absent from the duodenal bulb (uppermost region of duodenum), more prominent in the duodenum and jejunum, and gradually become less conspicuous in the terminal ileum. The mucosal surface area is further extended by finger-like projections called villi and depressions called crypts. There are 3 to 20 crypts surrounding each villus. The villi are 0.5 to 0.8 mm in height in the

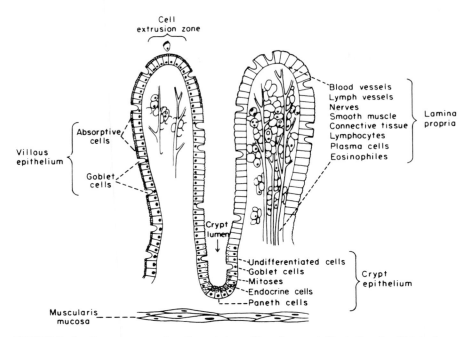

FIGURE 7–3. Transverse section through two villi and a crypt, illustrating the histologic organization of the small intestinal mucosa. (From Trier, J.S., and Modara, J.L.: Functional morphology of the mucosa of the small intestine. *In* Johnson, L.R. (ed.): Physiology of the Gastrointestinal Tract, Vol. II. New York, Raven Press, 1981, p. 926.)

duodenum and jejunum but rarely exceed 0.5 mm in the ileum. Crypt depth usually ranges between 0.3 and 0.6 mm. Finally, each villus and crypt is lined by columnar epithelial cells which, in turn, are covered with numerous closely packed microvilli. The microvilli on the cells at the tip of the villus (1.0 to 1.5 μm) are longer than those on the cells lining the crypts (0.5 μm). The combination of the plicae circulares, the villi, and the microvilli increases the mucosal surface area by about 600-fold (Fig. 7–2), creating a total surface area of 200 sq m. However, the effective area available for absorption is considerably less than this value owing to the closeness of adjacent villi and the inaccessibility of the lower two thirds of the villi and crypts to luminal contents.

Muscularis Mucosae

The mucosa of the small intestine can be subdivided into three distinct layers: the muscularis mucosae, the lamina propria, and the epithelium (Fig. 7–3). The base of the mucosa is lined by a thin continuous sheet of smooth muscle cells about 3 to 10 cells thick, separating the mucosa from the submucosa. This sheet of muscle is called the muscularis mucosae. Its physiologic functions are currently unknown; however, it may control the movement of villi.

Lamina Propria

The lamina propria consists primarily of connective tissue. It supports the epithelial lining, forming the core of each villus and surrounding the crypts. In addition to providing structural support, the lamina propria also contains blood vessels which nourish the epithelium and serve as conduits for transport of water-soluble substances absorbed by the epithelium. Within the core of the villus there is a large centrally located lymphatic vessel (the lacteal), which is the major channel for the transport of chylomicrons (lipids) to the systemic circulation. Some small unmyelinated nerve fibers, eosinophils, mast cells, fibroblasts, and smooth muscle cells are also present in the lamina propria. The smooth muscle cells are oriented along the longitudinal axis of the villus and presumably play a role in villus contractions.

There is mounting evidence that the lymphoid cells and associated structures of the lamina propria have important immunologic functions. Plasma cells, lymphocytes, and macrophages populate the lamina propria. In addition, small lymphoid nodules are present in the upper small intestine, while in the ileum large organized aggregates of lymphoid tissue (Peyer's patches) extend as deeply as the submucosa. Peyer's patches contain both B and T lymphocytes, as well as B cell precursors, which are destined to populate the lamina propria of the intestine. The lymphoid cells, nodules, and Peyer's patches of the lamina propria, along with the intraepithelial lymphocytes, constitute the so-called "gut-associated lymphoid tissue" or GALT. GALT is one of the major subdivisions of the immune system. Peyer's patches are considered to be the initiating sites of mucosal immunity, since they contain a precursor population of B lymphocytes that migrate to and populate the lamina propria. These cells in turn synthesize and secrete immunoglobulins (primarily IgA). GALT appears to be the first line of defense against enteric microbes and other antigenic material (e.g., food products).

Epithelium

A continuous sheet of epithelial cells (one cell thick) covers the surfaces of the villi and lines the crypts. The cell types which have been identified in the epithelial lining of the small intestine are listed in Table 7–1. Some of the cell types (e.g., goblet cells) are common to both villus and crypt epithelium, while others are exclusively found either in the villus region (e.g., enterocytes) or crypt region (e.g., undifferentiated cells).

The most prevalent cell type on the villus surface is the simple columnar absorptive cell, or enterocyte (Fig. 7–4). The most striking feature of the enterocyte is the presence of 3000 to 7000 microvilli on its apical surface. The plasma membrane covering the microvilli is coated with a filamentous glyco-

TABLE 7–1.   Epithelial Cells Lining the Villi and Crypts of the Small Intestine

Cell Type	Location	Function
Enterocytes	villus	digestion and absorption
Goblet cells	villus and crypt	mucus secretion
Endocrine cells	villus and crypt	hormone secretion
M cells	villus	absorption of food antigens
Intraepithelial lymphocytes	villus	unknown
Paneth cells	crypt	unknown
Caveolated cells	villus and crypt	unknown
Undifferentiated cells	crypt	precursor cells

protein-containing structure, the glycocalyx. The microvillus and its glycocalyx (the brush border) are viewed as the digestive-absorptive unit of the enterocyte. The plasma membrane of microvilli has an unusually large protein-to-lipid ratio, owing to the presence of specialized proteins possessing enzymatic, receptor, and transport properties. A number of enzymes involved in the hydrolysis of peptides (peptidases) and carbohydrates (disaccharidases) to transportable moieties (e.g., amino acids and glucose) are found in the microvillus membrane. In addition, proteins that are responsible for the co-transport of Na^+ and various organic solutes have been localized in the microvillus membranes. Finally, receptor proteins specific for certain substances have been localized to the microvilli of enterocytes in different regions of the small intestine. For example, the receptors for the intrinsic factor–vitamin B_{12} complex are present in the microvilli of ileal, but not jejunal, enterocytes, providing an explanation for why vitamin B_{12} absorption occurs exclusively in the ileum. The specific functions of the glycocalyx are not clear; it may provide a binding surface for absorption of pancreatic enzymes and offer support for large hydrophilic portions of intrinsic enzymes of the microvilli.

The basolateral membrane of the enterocyte is strikingly different from the apical "brush border" membrane. Its protein-to-lipid ratio is lower, and it is thinner and more permeable than the brush border membrane. The enzyme, Na^+,K^+-ATPase, is present at the basolateral membrane but not at the brush border. The fact that the Na^+,K^+-ATPase is limited to the basolateral membrane emphasizes the importance of this membrane in electrolyte transport.

In addition to the enterocytes, the mucosal epithelium contains secretory cells such as goblet cells and endocrine cells. These secretory cells are not limited to the villus (as are the enterocytes) but are also present in the crypts. The goblet cells secrete their product (mucus) into the lumen of the gut, whereas the secretions of the endocrine cells are directed into the lamina propria. These two secretory cells have different distribution frequencies along the gut. The goblet cells are more prevalent in the lower than in the upper small intestine, whereas the endocrine cells are generally more numerous in the upper portion of the gut.

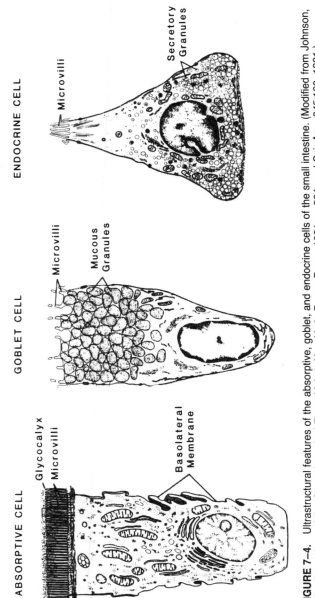
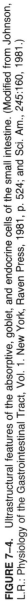

FIGURE 7–4.   Ultrastructural features of the absorptive, goblet, and endocrine cells of the small intestine. (Modified from Johnson, L.R.: Physiology of the Gastrointestinal Tract, Vol. 1. New York, Raven Press, 1981, p. 524; and Sci. Am., 245:160, 1981.)

Goblet cells are mucus-secreting cells that have a characteristic "wine goblet" appearance (Fig. 7–4). The apical portion of the cell is distended by many mucin-containing granules, while the nucleus and remaining cytoplasm are displaced to the narrow basal region. The luminal brush border is less developed than those of enterocytes, the microvilli being shorter and more sparsely distributed. The mucin granules are discharged into the lumen in response to noxious luminal stimuli (i.e., irritation) to form a protective coat of mucus over the epithelium.

The apical portion of the endocrine cell is narrow and contains tufts of microvilli which protrude into the lumen. These tufts are presumed to contain chemoreceptors which are sensitive to specific luminal stimuli. Some endocrine cells have a highly developed system of cytoplasmic filaments which serve to release hormones in response to mechanical stimuli. The distribution and secretory products of the more conventional endocrine cell types are shown in Figure 1–2 (see Chap. 1). Individual cells secrete either a peptide (e.g., cholecystokinin), or an amine (e.g., serotonin), or both (e.g., serotonin and substance P). Some of these cells have a true endocrine function, releasing their hormones to act at distant sites. Examples of these are the cells which store and secrete cholecystokinin, secretin, and GIP. Other endocrine cells appear to have a paracrine function, secreting hormones (somatostatin and serotonin) that modulate local events.

The mucosal epithelium contains two types of specialized cells that are part of the GALT system, the M cells and the intraepithelial lymphocytes. The M cells are interspersed among the enterocytes in the mucosal epithelium overlying the Peyer's patches. They are shaped like the letter **M**, with a thin apical portion bridging adjacent enterocytes and cytoplasmic extensions along the lateral margins of the enterocytes. The M cells usually envelop several lymphocytes and macrophages. Their apical portions are devoid of microvilli, being covered instead by a series of ridges one third to one fifth the height of the microvilli of enterocytes. The numerous pinocytotic vesicles located in the apical region of M cells suggests that these cells function to transport antigenic substances from the lumen to the intestinal lymphoid system. The intraepithelial lymphocytes are more ubiquitously distributed, accounting for about one sixth of the villus epithelium. They are larger than the simple lymphocytes of the lamina propria, but their specific function is not clear.

Two other cell types have been identified in the epithelium: the caveolated cells, which are dispersed throughout the villus and crypt regions, and the Paneth cells, which are confined to the crypts. The functional importance of these cells is unknown.

There is considerable evidence indicating that mature absorptive, goblet, endocrine, and Paneth cells are derived from undifferentiated cells lining the crypts. The undifferentiated cells are the most abundant cell type in the crypts and are extremely proliferative. Because of their high mitotic rate, these cells are extremely sensitive to radiation, ischemia, and antimitotic agents (methotrexate and colchicine). As they divide, the cells migrate up the crypt epithelium and differentiate into the different mature specialized cells that populate the villi. The best recognized aspect of this maturation process is the acquisition of the full complement of enzymes characteristic of the mature enterocyte, a gradual process which occurs as these cells migrate to the villus tip.

The absorptive, goblet, and endocrine cells continue to migrate up the villus until they arrive at the tip, from which they are extruded into the lumen. Normally, the villus cell population is maintained constant owing to a balance between cell exfoliation at the villus tips and proliferation and maturation of the cells in the crypts. The process of maturation, migration, and extrusion requires approximately 3 to 6 days. The cell turnover time is greater in the proximal than in the distal bowel, presumably owing to the greater height of villi in this region. The Paneth cells never leave the crypts; they eventually degenerate and are phagocytosed by cells lining the crypts. The turnover time for Paneth cells is several weeks.

The epithelium of the small intestine is a dynamic sheet of specialized cells governing the movement of materials between the lumen and the lamina propria. The most important function of the villus epithelium is the absorption of ingested nutrients and water, whereas the crypt epithelium serves as a source for the mature specialized cells of the villi.

Mucosal Growth and Adaptation

The high cell turnover rate of the small intestinal mucosa is closely regulated to maintain a balance between cell loss and cell production. Growth of the mucosa occurs when the turnover rate decreases, i.e., increased cell proliferation or decreased cell loss or both. Atrophy occurs when the turnover rate increases, i.e., decreased cell proliferation or increased cell loss or both. Mucosal growth is affected by several factors, all of which are linked to the presence of food in the gastrointestinal tract. It is well documented that food deprivation will cause a reduction in villus height and crypt depth. The starvation-induced atrophy can be reversed by oral, but not parenteral, feeding. The physiologic stress of lactation is associated with hypertrophy and hyperplasia of the intestinal mucosa. An increased food intake in response to the nutritional demands of lactation is believed to be the stimulus for mucosal growth. Intestinal resection induces an adaptive hyperplasia of the remaining intestinal mucosa. For example, resection of the jejunum leads to changes in the ileum, which now takes on the structural and functional characteristics of the jejunum. The postsurgical increase in mucosal mass occurs only if oral feeding, rather than parenteral feeding, is instituted. The mechanisms by which food intake induces adaptative growth in response to physiologic and surgical stresses are shown in Figure 7–5. The presence of food in the lumen can directly influence mucosal growth by providing nutrients for the mucosal cells; i.e., the enterocytes can derive nutritional support from absorbed material before the nutrients enter the circulation. In addition, luminal nutrients can initiate the release of gastrointestinal

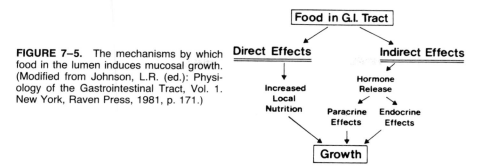

FIGURE 7–5. The mechanisms by which food in the lumen induces mucosal growth. (Modified from Johnson, L.R. (ed.): Physiology of the Gastrointestinal Tract, Vol. 1. New York, Raven Press, 1981, p. 171.)

hormones which regulate mucosal growth either by a paracrine or endocrine action. Gastrin, released from the antrum, has been implicated as the hormonal regulator of mucosal growth in the small intestine and in the functional development of the intestinal mucosa. Enteroglucagon has also been proposed as a mediator of intestinal growth.

WATER AND ELECTROLYTE ABSORPTION

Water Absorption

The small intestine of normal healthy individuals absorbs large quantities of water each day. This water is derived from ingested food and drink (approximately 1.0 to 1.5 liters per day) and from the secretions of the salivary glands, stomach, pancreas, liver, and intestine (approximately 6.0 to 7.0 liters per day). The total daily water load presented to the small intestine is roughly 8 liters and approximately 80 per cent of it is absorbed. The maximal absorptive capacity of the small intestine is unknown but may be as high as 15 liters per day. In some animals (e.g., rat, cow), water absorption can proceed at such a rapid rate that intravascular hemolysis occurs.

Water transport in the small intestine is passive, with the rate of absorption varying with the location along the bowel (duodenum or ileum), the rate of active solute transport, and luminal osmolality. The duodenum and jejunum are the major sites of water absorption, which can be explained by the relatively large pore size (8 Å, radius) and consequent low resistance to water movement across their mucosae. Water movement across the ileal mucosa is more restricted due to the existence of smaller pores (4 Å).

Water can move with facility either into or out of the intestinal lumen, depending upon the total osmotic activity of intestinal contents. Thus, the direction and magnitude of water movement in the proximal bowel are largely influenced by the nature of the ingested meal. Ingestion of a *hypotonic* meal (approximately 200 mOsm) leads to net water flow from intestinal lumen to blood, with the blood-lumen osmotic pressure difference acting as the driving force (Fig. 7–6). Water leaves the lumen more rapidly than electrolytes and

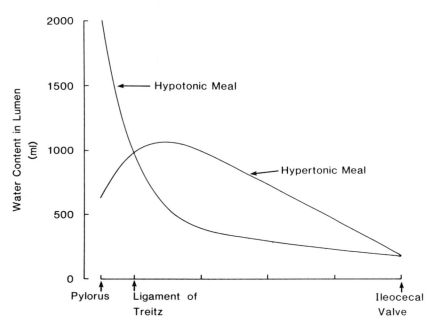

FIGURE 7–6. Water content in lumen along the small intestine after a hypotonic (steak) meal and a hypertonic (doughnut-milk) meal. (Adapted from Fordtran, J.S., and Ingelfinger, F.J. *In* Code, C.F., and Heidel, W. (eds.): Alimentary Canal. III. Intestinal Absorption. Baltimore, Williams and Wilkins, 1968.)

absorbable nutrients; therefore, luminal osmolality rises until it equals plasma osmolality. Ingestion of a *hypertonic* meal (approximately 600 mOsm) leads to net water movement from blood to bowel lumen. The accumulation of water in the lumen, and the movement of ions and nutrients out of the lumen, leads to dilution of chyme and brings the luminal contents to isotonicity. As illustrated in Figure 7–6, the distal small bowel plays a more important role in the absorption of water and electrolytes following a hypertonic meal, while the proximal bowel is more important following hypotonic meals. The important physiologic aspect of water fluxes in the duodenum is that net movement of water is in the direction which maintains isotonicity of the intestinal contents with plasma. The transfer of water by osmosis to make chyme isosmotic with plasma requires only a few minutes (50 per cent is absorbed in 3 minutes). Thereafter, the chyme remains isosmotic during its passage through the small intestine.

The net flow of water across the intestinal mucosa is the result of two large unidirectional fluxes. One flux is directed from the intestinal lumen to the interstitial fluid and then to blood or lymph vessels. The second flux occurs in the opposite direction, i.e., from interstitial fluid to lumen. The difference between the blood-to-lumen (secretory) and lumen-to-blood (absorptive) fluxes represents the net water flux. The magnitude of the net water flux in the small bowel is one fifth to one tenth that of the two unidirectional fluxes. For example:

$$\frac{\text{Net water flux}}{\text{(ml/min)}} = (\text{Lumen-to-blood flux}) - (\text{Blood-to-lumen flux})$$

$$0.20 = 2.20 \qquad\qquad\qquad - 2.00$$

As a result of the large difference between net and unidirectional fluxes, a relatively small change in one of the unidirectional fluxes has a great impact on net water movement. Alterations of the unidirectional water fluxes account for the rapid attainment of osmotic equilibrium of chyme entering the duodenum. Hypotonic chyme enhances the lumen-to-blood flux of water, thereby inducing net water absorption. Conversely, hypertonic chyme can cause net water secretion by enhancing the blood-to-lumen flux. When luminal osmolality exceeds plasma osmolality by 100 to 130 mOsm, the two unidirectional fluxes are equal, and the net flux of water is zero. Further increments in lumen osmolality lead to net water secretion.

While the rate of water absorption in the duodenum is highly dependent upon lumen osmolality, water movement across the mucosa of distal segments of the bowel is more closely coupled to solute transport, because here the lumen is in osmotic equilibrium with plasma. The coupling of solute and water fluxes in the jejunum and ileum can be explained by the standing osmotic gradient theory. According to this model, an osmotic gradient is established between the lumen and lateral intercellular space by active transport of electrolytes into the latter compartment. The osmotic gradient draws water across the tight junction and through the cell into the intercellular space. Therefore, as ions are absorbed so is an isosmotic equivalent of water. Because the mucosal membrane of the ileum offers more resistance to water movement (due to the small pores), the composition of absorbed fluid is slightly hypertonic in this region of the small bowel.

Electrolyte Absorption

SODIUM

The small intestine functions as a highly efficient sodium-conserving organ. The average adult intake of sodium is approximately 250 to 300 mEq per day. A similar amount of sodium enters the intestinal lumen from salivary, gastric, biliary, pancreatic, and intestinal secretions. Only 1 to 5 mEq of sodium is excreted in the stool; therefore, over 95 per cent of the sodium load entering the small bowel is eventually absorbed. Over half of the sodium is absorbed in the jejunum and, of the remainder, half is absorbed in the ileum and the rest in the colon. The rates of sodium absorption in the human jejunum and ileum are essentially the same, but the predominant mechanism of transport is different.

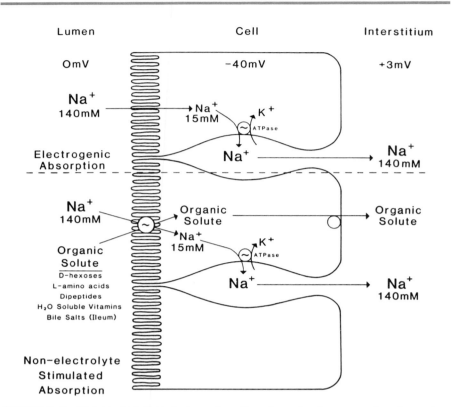

FIGURE 7–7. Cellular models of electrogenic sodium absorption (upper panel) and non-electrolyte stimulated absorption (lower panel) in the small intestine.

Several mechanisms are responsible for sodium absorption in the small intestine. These include (1) electrogenic (uncoupled) sodium absorption, (2) nonelectrolyte-stimulated sodium absorption, (3) neutral sodium chloride absorption, and (4) passive (convective) sodium absorption. Electrogenic sodium absorption involves an active process in which sodium movement is not directly coupled to the movement of other solutes (Fig. 7–7). Sodium entry into the cell is a result of simple diffusion down both concentration and electrical potential gradients. A basolateral sodium pump (Na^+,K^+-ATPase) provides the driving force for sodium extrusion from the epithelial cell. Sodium exit from the cell is directed against steep chemical (15 mM to 140 mM) and electrical (-40 mv to $+3$ mv) gradients. The energy required for this "uphill" transport is derived from ATP hydrolysis via the Na^+,K^+-ATPase. Because the sodium pump extrudes three sodium ions for every two potassium ions, a potential difference is created (an electrogenic potential) between the cell interior and exterior. Transport of sodium out of the cell at the basolateral membrane serves to maintain a low intracellular sodium concentration and a negative electrical potential, thus providing the electrochemical driving force for sodium entry into the cell. Ouabain, an inhibitor of Na^+,K^+-ATPase, abolishes electrogenic sodium absorption.

The absorption of a wide variety of water-soluble compounds in the small intestine is coupled to sodium absorption (Fig. 7–7). This mechanism of sodium transport is referred to as nonelectrolyte-stimulated sodium absorption. According to this model, a carrier molecule in the brush border membrane couples the entry of sodium and an organic solute (e.g., glucose) into the cell. As with electrogenic sodium absorption, sodium is extruded from the cell via the basolateral sodium pump (Na^+,K^+-ATPase), thereby creating an electrochemical gradient for sodium entry into the cell. The movement of sodium along its electrochemical gradient indirectly provides energy for the movement of the organic solute against its concentration gradient, i.e., from gut lumen into the cell. Extrusion of the organic solute out of the cell is directed down a concentration gradient and results from carrier-mediated facilitated diffusion.

Neutral sodium chloride absorption is a process whose net effect is one-for-one transport of sodium and chloride from gut lumen to plasma (Fig. 7–8). Two models have been proposed to explain neutral NaCl absorption in the small intestine. One model invokes a carrier molecule (comparable to non-electrolyte-stimulated absorption) which couples the entry of sodium and chloride at the brush border membrane. The energetics of uphill chloride transport into the cell are provided by the sodium gradient; i.e., extrusion of sodium across the basolateral membrane provides energy for uphill transport of chloride by maintaining a low intracellular sodium concentration. Sodium is transported out of the cell via the Na^+,K^+-ATPase activated pump, while chloride ions passively diffuse out of the cell along their electrochemical gradient.

Another model used to explain neutral NaCl absorption invokes the existence of two neutral countertransport processes: a sodium-hydrogen exchange process and a chloride-bicarbonate exchange process (Fig. 7–8). According to this model, water reacts with carbon dioxide in the epithelial cell, in the presence of carbonic anhydrase, to form carbonic acid, which in turn dissociates into hydrogen and bicarbonate ions. The "downhill" movement of sodium into the cell indirectly provides energy for the "uphill" movement of hydrogen ions from cell interior into the lumen. Likewise, the "downhill" transport of bicarbonate ions out of the cell energizes the "uphill" entry of chloride into the cell. The hydrogen and bicarbonate ions that enter the lumen rapidly form water and carbon dioxide; therefore, the net effect of this process is one-for-one absorption of sodium chloride. Neutral sodium chloride absorption may be regulated by cyclic AMP and calcium, since an increase in the intracellular concentration of either substance inhibits this absorptive process.

Another mechanism of sodium absorption in the small intestine is passive transport secondary to bulk flow of water. This process is of greater importance in the jejunum because of the relatively large size of pores in the mucosal membrane. Studies of the human jejunum suggest that as much as 85 per cent

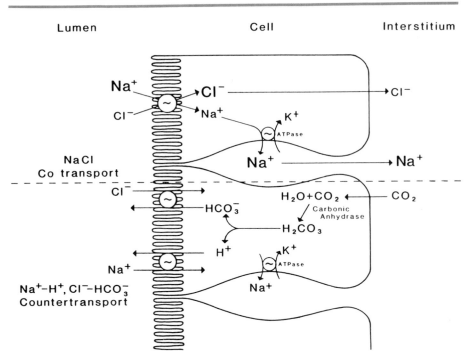

FIGURE 7–8. Cellular models of neutral sodium chloride absorption. The upper panel depicts a sodium chloride cotransport mechanism, while a sodium-hydrogen, chloride-bicarbonate countertransport process is illustrated in the lower panel.

of the enhanced sodium transport during glucose absorption is passive, with the active transport of glucose carrying sodium along with the absorbed water (convection). Passive absorption of sodium by convection occurs largely through the lateral spaces and tight junctions (which are twice as permeable to sodium and potassium as to chloride) with little transcellular movement. Passive sodium absorption secondary to convection is minimal in the ileum with its relatively small pores.

While all of the aforementioned mechanisms for sodium absorption are operative along the entire small bowel, the relative contribution of each process to total sodium transport differs in the jejunum and ileum. Passive (convective) sodium transport is the predominant process in the jejunum, with a lesser contribution made by electrogenic and nonelectrolyte-stimulated sodium absorption. In the ileum, electrogenic sodium absorption and neutral sodium chloride absorption are predominant, with minimal contributions from non-electrolyte-stimulated absorption and passive (convective) transport.

POTASSIUM

The average daily adult intake of potassium is 40 to 60 mEq. Most of the ingested potassium is absorbed in the jejunum, with little absorption taking place in the ileum. Potassium absorption in the jejunum is largely passive, with diffusion occurring down a concentration gradient (lumen-to-plasma) of approximately 10 mEq per liter (14 mEq/liter in lumen and 4 mEq/liter in plasma). Diffusion of potassium across the jejunal mucosa occurs primarily through the lateral spaces and tight junctions.

CHLORIDE

Intestinal absorption of chloride ions involves both active and passive processes. In the jejunum, chloride absorption is primarily passive, with both electrical and concentration gradients acting as driving forces. Potential difference–sensitive chloride absorption results from the small (3 to 5 mv) positive electrical potential between the gut lumen and plasma created by active sodium (coupled and uncoupled) transport. Concentration-dependent chloride absorption occurs when the luminal chloride ion concentration exceeds 100 mEq per liter (plasma). The diffusional flow (down both concentration and potential difference gradients) of chloride ions occurs largely through the lateral spaces and tight junctions and serves to maintain electrical neutrality across the jejunal mucosa. Chloride absorption in the ileum is active and results primarily from the neutral sodium chloride absorptive process described above (Fig. 7–8). The ileum can absorb chloride ions against a concentration gradient of 40 to 50 mEq per liter. Chloride absorption is competitively inhibited by other halides (e.g., bromide) in the intestinal lumen. Of the 36 mEq of chloride entering the small bowel each day, only 2 mEq are excreted in the stool.

BICARBONATE

Bicarbonate is rapidly absorbed in the jejunum by a process which involves the formation of carbon dioxide from bicarbonate ions in chyme with hydrogen ions secreted by the mucosa. The reaction gives rise to a markedly elevated P_{CO_2} ($\sim$ 100 mm Hg), thereby providing a steep gradient for carbon dioxide diffusion into the mucosal epithelium. Within the cell, carbon dioxide reacts with water in the presence of carbonic anhydrase to form carbonic acid, which dissociates into hydrogen and bicarbonate ions. The bicarbonate ions diffuse into the blood while the hydrogen ions are secreted into the lumen. In the ileum, on the other hand, bicarbonate ions are actively secreted into the lumen in exchange for chloride ions (Fig. 7–8). As a result of this ion exchange process, the ileal contents become alkaline (pH between 7 and 8). Bicarbonate ions are also secreted into the lumen of the duodenum by the Brunner's glands. The alkaline secretion of the duodenal glands aids in the neutralization of acidic chyme from the stomach. The maximal bicarbonate output of the Brunner's

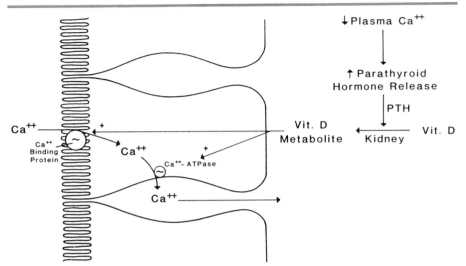

FIGURE 7–9. Mechanism of calcium absorption in the enterocytes of the small bowel. The vitamin D metabolite, 1,25 dihydroxycholecalciferol, stimulates calcium transport at both the apical and basolateral membranes.

glands is equivalent to basal pancreatic bicarbonate secretion. Secretin, which promotes bicarbonate delivery into the duodenum from both the pancreas and biliary system, also stimulates Brunner's gland secretion. Since carbonic anhydrase plays a primary role in bicarbonate absorption (jejunum) and secretion (duodenum, ileum), drugs which inhibit the enzyme block bicarbonate transport.

CALCIUM

Adult man ingests approximately 1.0 gram of calcium per day, half of which is from milk and milk products. An additional 200 to 300 mg are secreted into the intestine in various digestive juices. Most calcium is ingested in a nonionic form (e.g., calcium carbonate), which is insoluble at a neutral pH. However, gastric acid solubilizes the calcium salts and permits their absorption in the intestine. Approximately 40 per cent of the calcium entering the small bowel is absorbed. The duodenum and proximal jejunum are the primary sites of calcium absorption, with little if any calcium transport in the ileum. The uptake of calcium from the lumen is active when the luminal concentration is less than that of plasma (5 mEq per liter). At higher luminal concentrations, additional absorption takes place by simple diffusion. Active calcium absorption involves a two-step process: (1) facilitated diffusion or active transport into the cell and (2) active transport out of the cell (Fig. 7–9). The second step is the slower one and is, therefore, rate-limiting. Entry of calcium into the cell is modulated by a calcium-binding protein in the brush border membrane. Extrusion of calcium from the cell takes place at the basolateral membrane and involves a Ca^{++}-ATPase activated pump.

The rate of intestinal calcium absorption is controlled by an indirect negative feedback system involving the extracellular calcium concentration, a metabolite of vitamin D produced by the kidney (1,25-dihydroxycholecalciferol), and parathyroid hormone. Both steps involved in active calcium absorption are influenced by the blood concentration of 1,25-dihydroxycholecalciferol. The vitamin D metabolite enhances the synthesis of calcium-binding protein, the concentration of which correlates closely with the rate of calcium transport. Parathyroid hormone (PTH) exerts significant influence on intestinal calcium absorption by increasing the rate of conversion of vitamin D to 1,25-dihydroxycholecalciferol in the kidney. Feedback regulation of calcium absorption occurs as follows (Fig. 7–9): a reduction in the extracellular calcium concentration stimulates the release of PTH from the parathyroid gland, which in turn enhances the conversion of vitamin D to its active metabolite in the kidney. The vitamin D metabolite directly enhances intestinal calcium absorption, thereby restoring the extracellular calcium concentration to its normal value. Because of the time required for synthesis of calcium binding protein, there is a 3- to 5-hour delay in the effect of PTH on intestinal calcium absorption.

MAGNESIUM

Approximately 0.4 to 0.5 gram of magnesium is ingested each day by the adult human. Of this amount, about one third is absorbed in the small intestine. Absorption occurs along the entire length of the bowel with higher rates of transport in the proximal segments. The mechanism of magnesium transport appears to be passive, i.e., simple diffusion and convection.

IRON

The average daily intake of iron is 10 to 20 mg. In the carnivorous diet, iron is ingested mainly in the form of myoglobin and hemoglobin. Iron is released from digested food by the action of hydrochloric acid and proteolytic enzymes in the stomach. Ferric (Fe^{+++}) ions are reduced to the ferrous (Fe^{++}) state by ascorbic acid in the diet. Within the small bowel, the ferrous ion is bound to molecules such as ascorbic acid, citric acid, amino acids, sugars, and alcohol, which increase its solubility and, consequently, its absorption. Conversely, iron complexed with phytate, oxalate, and phosphates is relatively insoluble and is poorly absorbed. Approximately 10 per cent of the total iron entering the small intestine is absorbed, while menstruating females absorb a greater amount.

The major sites of iron absorption are the duodenum and proximal jejunum. Iron enters the intestinal epithelium either as heme or an inorganic ion, with the ferrous form more rapidly absorbed than the ferric, and heme-iron more readily absorbed than inorganic iron. Heme-iron is transported as heme into

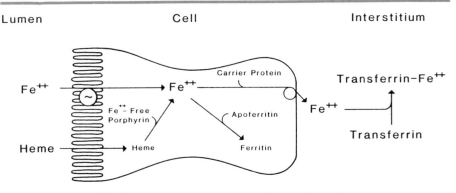

FIGURE 7–10.   Iron absorption in the small intestine.

the cell where it is split by a heme-splitting enzyme (which is linked to xanthine oxidase) to ferrous ion and iron-free porphyrin (Fig. 7–10). Once the ferrous ion is released in the cytoplasm it is either transported, via a protein carrier, to the serosal aspect of the cell where it is extruded by an active process, or it combines with apoferritin to form ferritin, which sequesters the iron within the cell as ferric micelles. Ferrous ions in the lumen are actively transported into the cell at the brush border and then follow one of the two pathways noted above for heme-iron. The serosal transfer and extrusion of ferrous ions is a slower process than the uptake of heme and ferrous ions at the brush border; therefore, the serosal step is rate-limiting in the regulation of iron absorption. Once iron is extruded from the epithelial cell, it binds with transferrin, a plasma protein which transports the ion to other tissues.

The rate of iron release from intestinal epithelia to plasma is largely governed by the need for iron in body tissues (Fig. 7–11). Iron deficiency is associated with an increased transfer of iron from intestinal lumen to plasma, while during iron overload there is decreased transfer. Two theories have been proposed to explain feedback regulation of intestinal iron absorption. According to one theory, the influence of body iron levels on iron absorption is mediated by crypt cell ferritin content. If the body iron stores are low, there is little stimulus for the synthesis of apoferritin and ferritin in the crypt cell. Thus, when the cell has migrated to the upper portion of the villus, there is relatively little ferritin, and most of the iron entering the cell is rapidly transferred to plasma. On the other hand, when body stores of iron are excessive, there is an increased synthesis of ferritin and apoferritin in the crypt cell. When these ferritin-rich cells reach the villus tips, most of the absorbed iron is sequestered in ferritin micelles, and very little iron is transported to the plasma. Within a few days the iron-loaded cell is sloughed off, and its complement of iron is lost in the feces. In support of this theory is the observation that there is a lag of several days for the increase in iron absorption to occur following an acute blood loss.

The other major theory describing feedback regulation of iron absorption

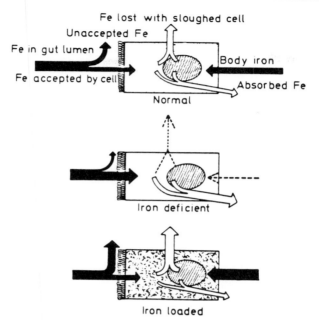

FIGURE 7–11.   Role of the intestinal mucosa in body iron regulation. Under normal conditions iron enters the cell from both the lumen and the plasma. Part of absorbed iron and iron derived from the plasma is stored as ferritin. As the cells are sloughed at the villus tips, iron is lost into the lumen. In the iron-deficient individual more iron is absorbed from the lumen and a smaller fraction of the absorbed iron is stored as ferritin. Therefore, less iron is lost with sloughed cells. In the iron-loaded individual there is a reduction in iron absorption, yet ferritin becomes saturated with iron derived from the plasma. With cell sloughing there is a greater loss of iron into the lumen. (From Conrad, M.E., Jr., and Crosby, W.H.: Intestinal mucosal mechanisms controlling iron absorption. Blood, 22:406, 1963.)

holds that the body stores of iron govern absorption by directly influencing the rate of uptake and extrusion of iron by the epithelial cell. In the iron-deficient state, there is rapid uptake of inorganic iron and heme, the activity of the heme iron-splitting enzyme is enhanced, and transport of iron within (via the carrier protein) and out of the cell is increased. The net effect is an increased transport of iron from intestinal lumen to blood. Conversely, with iron overload, cellular uptake and extrusion of iron is depressed, and there is a reduction of iron absorption.

SECRETION OF WATER AND ELECTROLYTES

Net water and electrolyte transport across the mucosa of the small intestine represents the difference between lumen-to-blood and blood-to-lumen fluxes. While the difference between the unidirectional fluxes normally favors net water absorption, it is estimated that 2 to 3 liters of isotonic fluid are secreted

TABLE 7–2.   Agents and Conditions Producing Net Fluid Secretion in the Small Intestine

Hormones and Neurotransmitters	
Glucagon	Acetylcholine
Secretin	Serotonin
Vasoactive intestinal polypeptide	Substance P
Prostaglandin E_1	Cholecystokinin
Bacterial Toxins	
Vibrio cholerae	*Staphylococcus aureus*
Escherichia coli	*Clostridium perfringens*
Bacillus cereus	*Pseudomonas aeruginosa*
Shigella dysenteriae	*Klebsiella pneumoniae*
Laxatives	
Ricinoleic acid (active ingredient of castor oil)	Phenolphthalein
Dihydroxy bile acids	Magnesium salts
Physical Factors	
Luminal distention	Increased luminal osmolality
Plasma dilution	Increased mucosal permeability
Increased interstitial hydrostatic pressure	

by the small intestine each day. The physiologic role of intestinal secretion remains unclear; however, its purpose may be to maintain the fluidity of chyme or to dilute potentially injurious substances or both, and to wash such substances away from the epithelial surface. It is now well recognized that excess stimulation of the normal secretory processes can create a disequilibrium between the absorptive and secretory water fluxes so that net fluid and electrolyte secretion and, ultimately, diarrhea result. Table 7–2 lists some of the many agents which stimulate water and electrolyte secretion in the small bowel. The water and electrolyte loss from patients with prolonged and severe diarrhea (e.g., choleragenic secretion) can result in dehydration of the body tissues and a severe electrolyte imbalance that can have rapidly fatal consequences (e.g., metabolic acidosis due to excess bicarbonate loss). Diarrheal disorders such as cholera are a leading cause of death worldwide, particularly in underdeveloped countries.

Secretion of water and electrolytes in the small intestine can be induced by the following mechanisms: active anion secretion, decreased solute absorption, increased luminal osmolality, and increased interstitial hydrostatic pressure. Active anion secretion has been demonstrated in the jejunum of normal human subjects. Several bacterial toxins, hormones, and detergents (e.g., bile acids) which induce net water secretion in the small bowel do so by stimulating active anion (chloride or bicarbonate) secretion. This process is mediated by a change in the intracellular cyclic AMP or calcium concentration or both, and it appears to be localized in the crypts of Lieberkühn. Accordingly, secretagogues such as cholera enterotoxin attach to specific receptors on the brush border membrane of crypt epithelium, which enhances adenyl cyclase activity, and thereby increases intracellular cAMP content. The rise in cAMP concentration then leads to solute-coupled fluid secretion into the intestinal (crypt) lumen. The fluid secreted by the crypts is usually alkaline and composed largely of isosmotic sodium chloride and bicarbonate. The concept that active secretory and absorptive processes in the intestine are spatially separated (the former in the crypts and the latter in the villi) has led to the notion that there is a continuous circulation of fluid from the crypts to the villi. Such a circulation of fluid may serve to minimize the thickness of stagnant water layers and propel secreted substances (e.g., immunoglobulins) out of the crypts toward the tips of the villi.

Another mechanism by which cholera enterotoxin produces net secretion of water and electrolytes is by inhibition of neutral sodium-chloride absorption in villus cells. The influence of cholera toxin on neutral sodium-chloride absorption also appears to be mediated by a rise in villus cell cAMP content. Because cholera toxin (and cAMP) does not inhibit glucose-stimulated sodium absorption, ingestion of glucose-electrolyte solutions has proven to be an effective therapeutic means of reducing the fluid loss in patients with cholera. Other secretagogues which exert all or part of their effect by inhibiting neutral sodium-chloride absorption include VIP, prostaglandin E_1, and theophylline.

Increased luminal osmolality is the primary mechanism responsible for net fluid secretion in the proximal small bowel of normal individuals. As discussed above, when hypertonic chyme enters the duodenal lumen from the stomach, the blood-to-lumen water flux increases in order to keep the luminal contents isotonic, and net fluid secretion results. Osmotic equilibration in the small intestine is also the basis of action of some laxatives. Magnesium sulfate is a poorly absorbed salt, and therefore it must retain its osmotic equivalent of water in the intestinal lumen either by preventing water absorption or by inducing water secretion (passive). A clinical example of luminal osmolality as a mechanism for net fluid secretion is the diarrhea associated with lactase deficiency. In this condition, an increased blood-to-lumen water flux results from the increased luminal osmotic pressure arising from lactose retention in the lumen (see Fig. 7–15).

Net water and electrolyte secretion can also be induced by an increase in the hydrostatic pressure gradient across the mucosal membrane. This type of secretion is commonly referred to as "secretory filtration" because it denotes the filtration of interstitial fluid into the bowel lumen. Secretory filtration does not occur across the mucosal membrane of the normal villus for two reasons: a low interstitial hydrostatic pressure (0 to 2 mm Hg) and a high resistance to water movement (low hydraulic conductance). Conditions (e.g., portal hypertension, plasma dilution) which greatly enhance capillary fluid filtration and lead to interstitial fluid accumulation produce a rise in interstitial hydrostatic pressure. When interstitial hydrostatic pressure increases to 4 to 6 mm Hg, the mucosal membrane ruptures at the villus tips, producing a one-thousandfold increase in mucosal hydraulic conductance. The decreased mucosal resistance to water flow, coupled to the rise in interstitial hydrostatic pressure, can lead to secretory filtration. A clinical example of secretory filtration may be the net

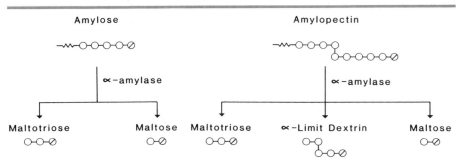

FIGURE 7–12. Major polysaccharides of starch and their hydrolytic products after exposure to α-amylase. Reducing glucose units are indicated by ø.

fluid secretion that is seen in the obstructed bowel, where luminal distention compresses the venous drainage and greatly enhances intestinal capillary filtration rate. It is uncertain, however, whether secretory filtration accounts for any part of normal fluid secretion by the small intestine.

CARBOHYDRATE DIGESTION AND ABSORPTION

Dietary Carbohydrates

Carbohydrates are an inexpensive source of calories worldwide. The principal dietary carbohydrates are starches, sucrose, and lactose. Approximately 400 gm of carbohydrates per day are consumed by humans in the Western world. Sixty per cent of the digestible carbohydrates is ingested in the form of starch, 30 per cent as sucrose, and 10 per cent as lactose. Indigestible carbohydrates, which are the main constituents of dietary fiber, account for a relatively small fraction of the Western diet.

Starch is a glucose-containing polysaccharide having a molecular weight of 100,000 to more than 1 million. The two major polysaccharides of starch are amylose and amylopectin (Fig. 7–12). Amylose is a straight chain of α 1,4-linked glucose molecules and it accounts for approximately 20 per cent of dietary starch. Amylopectin, accounting for 80 per cent of dietary starch, differs from amylose in that there are α 1,6-linkages approximately every 25 glucose molecules along the straight (α 1,4) chain. Glycogen, a high molecular weight polysaccharide found in animal tissues, is similar to amylopectin; however, the α 1,6-branch points occur with greater frequency, i.e., every 12 glucose residues.

Digestion

The initial step in the digestion of starch involves the hydrolysis of α 1,4-linkages by salivary and pancreatic α-amylases (Fig. 7–12). Salivary and pan-

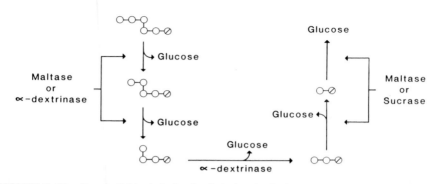

FIGURE 7–13. Sequential hydrolysis of α-limit dextrins by brush border oligosaccharidases. Reducing glucose units are indicated by ø. (From Gray, G.M.: Assimilation of dietary carbohydrate. Viewpoints Dig. Dis., *12:*3, 1980.)

creatic α-amylase exhibit optimal activity at near neutral pH. Thus, little starch hydrolysis occurs under the influence of the salivary α-amylase because of the short exposure time before gastric acid inactivates the enzyme. However, when food is chewed for an extended period of time, up to 75 per cent of the starch can be digested to the disaccharide stage by salivary α-amylase.

Intraluminal digestion of carbohydrates in the duodenum is extremely rapid because of the tremendous amount of amylase secreted by the pancreas. The final oligosaccharide products of luminal digestion are formed before a starch meal reaches the jejunum. Some pancreatic α-amylase is adsorbed to the brush border membrane of the mucosa where it hydrolyzes starch exposed to the surface of epithelial cells.

As an endoenzyme, α-amylase preferentially cleaves the interior 1,4-linkages and has very low specificity for the outermost links of the molecule. α-Amylase is incapable of cleaving the β 1,4-glucose linkages in cellulose, and it cannot break the α 1,6-branching links of amylopectin and glycogen. Consequently, the final hydrolytic products of α-amylase action on amylose are maltose (glucose-glucose, α 1,4-linkage) and maltotriose (glucose-glucose-glucose, α 1,4-linkages) (Fig. 7–12). Maltose (disaccharide) and maltotriose (trisaccharide) are also products of amylase action on amylopectin and glycogen. Branched oligosaccharides (with an average of 6 to 8 glucose units) containing both α 1,6- and α 1,4-linkages, which are known as α-limit dextrins, are also products of amylolytic digestion of amylopectin and glycogen (Fig. 7–12). α-Limit dextrins are formed owing to the fact that the α 1,6-linkages in amylopectin and glycogen are resistant to hydrolysis by α-amylase.

The products of luminal starch digestion and the other dietary sugars (sucrose and lactose) must be hydrolyzed to their monosaccharide constituents, because there are no mucosal transport mechanisms for saccharides having two or more hexose units (Fig. 7–13). The enzymes responsible for the complete hydrolysis of oligosaccharides are glycoproteins, which are an integral part of

TABLE 7–3.   Surface Hydrolysis of Oligosaccharides

Enzyme	Substrates	Molecular Site of Hydrolysis	Products
Maltase	Maltose, maltotriose	α-1,4 linkage	glucose
Sucrase*	Sucrose	α-1,4 linkage	glucose, fructose
Lactase	Lactose	β-1,4 linkage (but not of cellulose)	glucose, galactose
α-Dextrinase (isomaltase)	α-Limit dextrins	α-1,6 linkage	glucose, maltose, oligosaccharides

*Sucrase is also very active against maltose and maltotriose.

the brush border membrane and are positioned in it so that the active hydrolytic site is on the luminal surface of the membrane. Thus, their oligosaccharide substrates are hydrolyzed when they contact the brush border membrane. The activity of the mucosal membrane oligosaccharidases is highest in the mid-jejunum and lowest in the duodenum and terminal ileum.

The major brush border membrane oligosaccharidases are maltase, sucrase (also called invertase), lactase, and α-dextrinase (also called isomaltase). The substrates and products of each of the enzymes are summarized in Table 7–3. Maltase, the most active of the disaccharidases, hydrolyzes maltose and maltotriose to glucose. Sucrase is primarily involved in the hydrolysis of sucrose to its monosaccharide subunits, glucose and fructose, but it is also very active against maltose and maltotriose. Lactase, the least active of the disaccharidases, catalyzes the hydrolysis of lactose to glucose and galactose. The essential physiologic function of α-dextrinase is hydrolysis of α 1,6-linkages in α-limit dextrins; however, the enzyme is also capable of removing α 1,4-linked glucose residues from the nonreducing end of α-dextrins. As illustrated in Figure 7–13, the α-limit dextrins are hydrolyzed by the complimentary action of maltase and α-dextrinase, each of which acts at discrete regions on the oligosaccharide.

The activity of membrane-bound oligosaccharidases in the small bowel is so high that the absorption of hexoses, rather than hydrolysis of oligosaccharides, is the rate-limiting step in the overall assimilation of most carbohydrates. An exception to this is lactose, whose rate of hydrolysis by lactase is slower than the rate of absorption of its monosaccharide constituents. (Maltose is hydrolyzed as rapidly as sucrose, but lactose is cleaved only half as quickly.) The activity of the brush border oligosaccharidases is influenced to some extent by the carbohydrate composition of the diet. Changing from a sucrose-deficient diet to a high-sucrose diet leads to a doubling of sucrase and maltase activities within 2 to 5 days. Oligosaccharidase activities are not increased by diets rich in either lactose, maltose, or both.

Transport of Monosaccharides

The principal final products of surface hydrolysis of oligosaccharides are glucose, galactose, and fructose. Once the monosaccharides are released by surface digestion, either they diffuse a small distance to transport sites (carrier proteins) located very near the brush border enzyme, or they diffuse into the lumen to be absorbed by intestinal cells located more distally. The monosaccharides are too large to cross the mucosal membrane by simple diffusion to a significant degree. Therefore, specific carrier-mediated processes exist to ensure adequate absorption of glucose, galactose, and fructose. It is estimated that the human small intestine can absorb an amount of hexoses equivalent to 22 pounds of sucrose daily.

The aldohexoses, glucose and galactose, have a nearly identical structure and therefore share a single transport process (protein carrier). They are actively transported into the enterocyte by a process requiring energy and sodium. (Luminal sodium concentration is sufficiently high at all times not to limit the transport of the sugars.) A carrier molecule in the brush border membrane couples the entry of sodium and either glucose or galactose into the cell (Fig. 7–7). Sodium is extruded from the interior of the cell via the basolateral pump (Na^+,K^+-ATPase), thereby creating an electrochemical gradient for sodium entry into the cell. The movement of sodium along its electrochemical gradient indirectly provides energy for the movement of glucose (or galactose) against its concentration gradient, i.e., from gut lumen into the cell. A sodium-independent carrier molecule in the basolateral membrane transports most of the monosaccharide out of the cell by facilitated diffusion, and the remainder diffuses passively across the relatively porous basal regions of the cell. Energy for the aldohexose carrier mechanism located at the brush border membrane is required only when the luminal glucose (or galactose) concentration is lower than that in the cell. Thus, aldohexose absorption probably occurs along a downhill gradient into the cells of the upper small intestine following a carbohydrate meal, while uphill (active) transport occurs in the lower jejunum and ileum, where the luminal concentrations fall below those in blood.

The active transport of either glucose or galactose is inhibited by the presence of the other aldohexose; i.e., the absorption of glucose depresses the rate at which galactose is absorbed and vice versa, indicating competition for a site on the carrier. Inasmuch as glucose has a greater affinity for the carrier site, its absorption depresses galactose transport more than galactose absorption depresses the transport of glucose. The structural specificity of the aldohexose carrier molecule is also demonstrated by the fact that modifications or substitutions at certain positions in the glucose or galactose molecule prevent their active transport.

Fructose, the ketohexose released from the hydrolysis of sucrose, is absorbed by facilitated diffusion. The carrier molecule for fructose at the brush border membrane cannot be energized to carry out active transport, and it is sodium-independent. In some animals, a large fraction of the fructose entering the enterocytes is metabolized to glucose, which subsequently exits the cell at the basolateral membrane. In man, intracellular conversion of fructose to glucose is minimal and of limited significance. The rate of fructose absorption in man is normally one sixth to one third of the rate of glucose absorption.

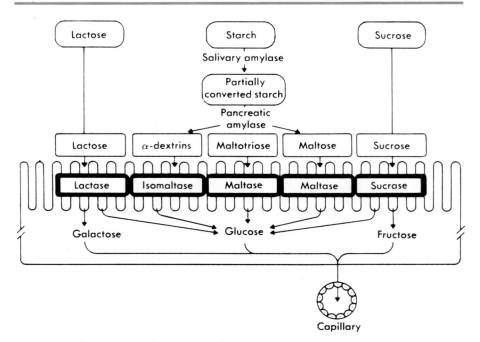

FIGURE 7–14. Summary of various steps involved in the assimilation of carbohydrates. (From Johnson, L.R.: Gastrointestinal Physiology. St. Louis, C.V. Mosby, 1981.)

Figure 7–14 summarizes the various steps involved in the assimilation of carbohydrates.

Carbohydrate Intolerance

Although pancreatic amylase–related maldigestion of starch is virtually nonexistent in the adult human (because the enzyme is secreted in great excess), deficiencies of membrane-bound disaccharidases are a frequent cause of carbohydrate malabsorption. The enzyme deficiency may be genetic or acquired, i.e., resulting from a disease of the small intestine such as celiac sprue (see Clinical Correlations). Lactase deficiency is the most common congenital disaccharidase deficiency, but it may also be acquired secondarily to intestinal disease. In the absence of lactase (or another disaccharidase), the unabsorbed disaccharide accumulates in the bowel lumen and increases luminal osmolality, which in turn draws water into the lumen by osmosis (Fig. 7–15). Metabolism of lactose by bacteria in the terminal ileum and colon leads to an increase in the number of osmotically active solutes in the lumen, thereby further increasing the osmotic effect of lactose. The end result of lactose accumulation (and metabolism) is an osmotic diarrhea. The patients complain of fullness and dis-

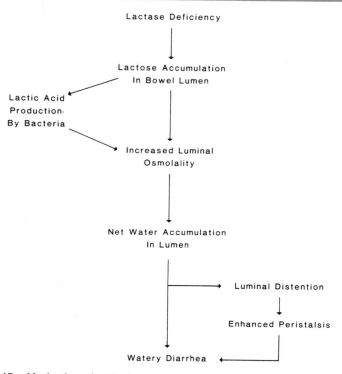

FIGURE 7–15. Mechanisms involved in excess water loss (diarrhea) produced by lactase deficiency (carbohydrate intolerance).

tention of the abdomen followed by increased flatus production (due to hydrogen and carbon dioxide gases produced by bacterial degradation of lactose) and watery diarrhea a few minutes to several hours after eating 10 to 50 grams of lactose. Primary lactase deficiency in adults is present in 5 to 20 per cent of whites and 70 to 75 per cent of blacks in North America. The deficiency is inherited as a dominant trait, and its symptoms can be eliminated by exclusion of dairy products from the diet.

Dietary Fiber

The term dietary fiber is generally used to describe the carbohydrate components of food that are not digested by the endogenous secretions of the human digestive tract. The major indigestible carbohydrates are cellulose, hemicelluloses, and pectins. A well-recognized characteristic of fiber is its ability to bind water, which explains why a high fiber diet increases the weight of the stool. Of all dietary factors, the fiber content of food seems to be the most important variable affecting mouth-to-anus transit time. The transit time decreases from approximately three days or longer for a low fiber diet to only

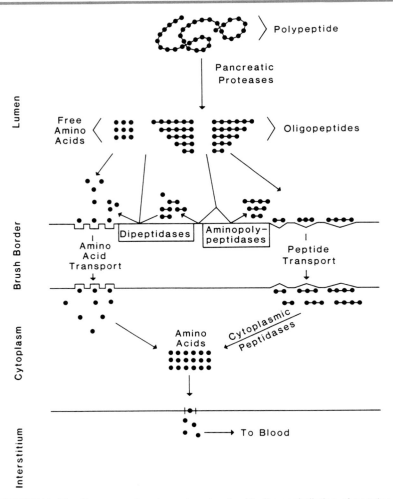

FIGURE 7–16. Summary of various steps involved in the assimilation of proteins.

20 to 30 hours for a high fiber diet. Inasmuch as dietary fiber adsorbs certain minerals (calcium, iron, magnesium, and zinc), there is a risk that excessive amounts of fiber in the diet may lead to mineral deficiencies. Severe zinc deficiencies have been described in populations whose diets include natural fibers as a major component. Dietary fiber also adsorbs organic materials such as bile salts and lipids. The absorption of lipid-soluble drugs and carcinogens by the bowel may be significantly reduced by a high fiber diet. The richest natural food sources of dietary fiber are the all-bran cereals, baked beans, peanut butter, and partially cooked peas, carrots, and potatoes.

PROTEIN DIGESTION AND ABSORPTION (Fig. 7–16)

Dietary Requirements

Unlike carbohydrate, protein is essential for growth of the young and the maintenance of health in adults. The protein content of the average American diet is 70 to 90 grams per day. The minimum daily protein intake required to achieve nitrogen balance ranges between 35 and 50 grams per day. Growing children and pregnant and lactating women require a proportionately greater protein intake relative to body weight to maintain nitrogen balance; i.e., young children require 4 grams per kg body weight per day, compared to 0.6 grams per kg body weight per day for adults. The proteins of the body are comprised of 20 different amino acids, only half of which can be synthesized in the body; the remainder (essential amino acids) must be provided in the diet. The dietary proteins are derived almost entirely from meats, fish, and vegetables. In general, meat and other animal proteins (e.g., milk, eggs) contain all of the essential amino acids, while vegetable proteins are deficient in one or more amino acids (e.g., zein, the protein of corn is deficient in lysine and tryptophan). Therefore, even if the daily intake of protein exceeds 35 to 50 grams, normal body growth is not likely to occur if the protein is derived from a single vegetable source.

Protein that is available for absorption in the small intestine is derived not only from food but also from digestive secretions (enzymes, mucoproteins), desquamated cells, and plasma proteins. Between 10 and 30 grams of protein per day enter the intestinal lumen via the digestive secretions, while epithelial shedding can produce as much as 50 grams per day. Although the intestinal mucosa is relatively impermeable to macromolecules, a significant quantity of plasma proteins enters the gut lumen each day. It is estimated that approximately 15 per cent of the normal turnover of albumin and γ-globulin can be accounted for by enteric protein loss, i.e., 3 grams per day. Thus, the proteins of endogenous origin nearly double the total amount of protein presented to the intestine for digestion and absorption. In spite of the large amounts of protein presented daily to the small intestine, less than 10 per cent escapes absorption and is lost in the stool.

Digestion

The complete digestion of proteins to amino acids requires a larger number of enzymes than is needed to reduce starch or fat to their constituent components. The first enzyme involved in the hydrolysis of protein is pepsin, which is secreted as pepsinogen from the chief cells of the gastric mucosa (see Chap. 4). When the stomach contents reach the duodenum, alkaline pancreatic juice causes the cessation of peptic activity. The extent of gastric protein digestion is determined by the physical state of the ingested protein (type of protein and extent of mastication), the activity of pepsin in gastric juice, and the length of time that it stays in the stomach. Ingested protein is usually transported to the duodenum as a mixture of native protein, proteoses, peptones, polypeptides, and only a minute quantity of free amino acids. Therefore, the gastric phase of protein digestion is generally considered to be of little importance, relative to intestinal digestion, in the overall assimilation of protein. The nonessential nature of pepsin-mediated protein digestion is demonstrated by the fact that patients with achlorhydria (failure of the stomach to secrete acid and pepsinogen) exhibit no impairment of protein assimilation; i.e., they remain in nitrogen balance on normal protein diets.

LUMINAL DIGESTION

When ingested protein and the products of gastric protein digestion reach the duodenum, they are mixed with the proteolytic enzymes secreted by the pancreas. Secretion of pancreatic enzymes is enhanced when food is present in the duodenal lumen, an effect mediated by the hormone cholecystokinin. The proteolytic enzymes of the pancreas are secreted as inactive precursors (proenzymes), which are subsequently activated in the duodenum (Fig. 7–17). Intraluminal activation involves the conversion of trypsinogen (inactive precursor) to trypsin (active protease), a reaction catalyzed by an endopeptidase released from enterocytes that is called "enterokinase." The presence of trypsin in the lumen further enhances its own formation (from trypsinogen), as well as activating the other peptidase precursors from the pancreas.

The proteolytic enzymes produced by the pancreas can be classified as either endopeptidases (trypsin, elastase, chymotrypsin) or exopeptidases (carboxypeptidases A and B). Endopeptidases act on specific peptide bonds at the interior of the protein molecule. For example, trypsin hydrolyzes only the peptide bonds formed by amino acids with a positively charged side chain (e.g., arginine, lysine), while chymotrypsin attacks only the peptide bonds formed by aromatic amino acids (e.g., tyrosine and phenylalanine). In contrast, the exopeptidases hydrolyze, in sequence, the carboxyl terminal peptide bond in the peptide chain. Intraluminal digestion of dietary protein occurs by sequential or essentially simultaneous action of the endo- and exopeptidases (Fig. 7–18). The endopeptidases yield oligopeptides that are ideal substrates for the exopeptidases, which in turn remove an amino acid from the carboxyl terminus of the peptide. The combined actions of the endopeptidases and exopeptidases result in a mixture of small peptides of two to six amino acid units and neutral and basic amino acids (particularly tyrosine, arginine, and methionine). The small peptides account for 70 per cent of the final products of intraluminal protein digestion, while the free amino acids account for the remainder. Inasmuch as the pancreas secretes a tremendous overabundance of proteolytic enzymes in response to a meal, membrane hydrolysis and absorption of small peptides (and amino acids) by the enterocytes, rather than intraluminal digestion, are the rate-limiting processes in overall protein assimilation.

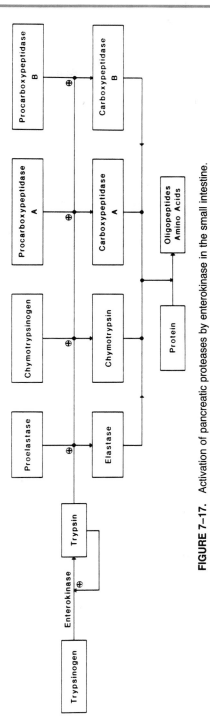

FIGURE 7–17. Activation of pancreatic proteases by enterokinase in the small intestine.

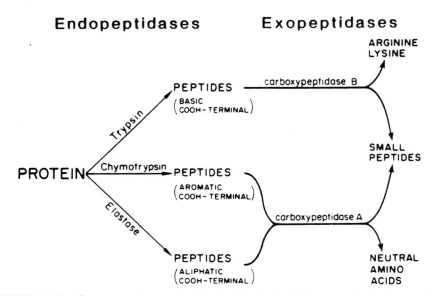

FIGURE 7–18. Sequence of events leading to hydrolysis of dietary protein by intraluminal proteases. (From Gray, G.M.: Mechanisms of digestion and absorption of food. *In* Sleisenger, M.H., and Fordtran, J.S. (eds.): Gastrointestinal Disease. Philadelphia, W.B. Saunders, 1983.)

CELLULAR DIGESTION OF PEPTIDES

The oligopeptides produced by pancreatic enzyme digestion are further hydrolyzed to free amino acids either at the surface of the brush border membrane or within the cytosol of the enterocyte. The site (brush border or cytosolic) of oligopeptide hydrolysis is largely determined by the number of amino acid residues in the peptide (Fig. 7–19). Specific carrier mechanisms exist at the brush border membrane which allow dipeptides and tripeptides to enter the cytoplasm of the enterocyte where they are hydrolyzed by specific peptidases (dipeptidase, amino-tripeptidase) to free amino acids. Oligopeptides with more than four amino acid residues either are not transported across the brush border membrane (e.g., hexapeptide) or are very poorly absorbed (e.g., tetrapeptide). Tetra- and higher (up to octapeptide) peptides are hydrolyzed by brush border peptidases (e.g., aminopolypeptidase) to di- and tripeptides and, to a lesser extent, free amino acids. The di- and tripeptides are then transported (by the aforementioned carrier mechanism) into the cytosol, where hydrolysis to amino acids is completed. Therefore, the end product of cellular peptide digestion is almost entirely free amino acids, which appear in portal blood after a protein meal.

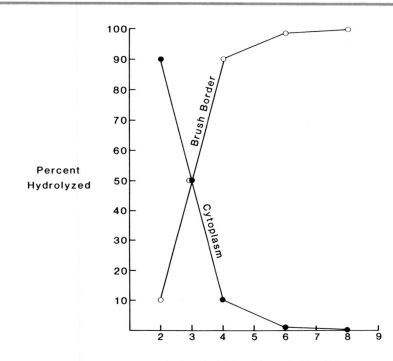

FIGURE 7–19.   Dependence of peptide hydrolysis by brush border and cytoplasmic peptidases on the number of amino acid residues in the peptide.

Peptide and Amino Acid Transport Mechanisms

PEPTIDES

Absorption of peptides is now considered to be the predominant mechanism for intestinal assimilation of dietary protein. It is well recognized that amino acids are absorbed at a much greater rate if introduced into the gut lumen as dipeptides and tripeptides rather than as free amino acids. Peptide absorption involves a carrier-mediated process which may be Na^+-dependent (see Fig. 7–7). The peptide transport mechanism shows a preference for dipeptides and tripeptides which contain glycine or proline residues. Tetrapeptides are transported to a limited extent. The peptide carriers transport both actively and passively, depending upon the luminal concentration of the peptide. Reducing the pH of intestinal chyme to 2, as with gastric hypersecretion, significantly depresses peptide absorption, while short-term (10 day) dietary restriction (50 per cent of normal intake) of protein increases the rate of peptide absorption.

TABLE 7–4.   Intestinal Amino Acid Transport Mechanisms

Mechanism	Amino Acids Transported	Type of Transport	Rate of Transport
Neutral	Aromatic (tyrosine, tryptophan, phenylalanine) Aliphatic (glycine*, alanine, serine, threonine, valine, leucine, isoleucine) Methionine, histidine, glutamine, asparagine, cysteine	Active, Na$^+$-dependent	Very rapid
Dibasic	Lysine, arginine, ornithine, cystine	Active, Na$^+$-dependent	Rapid (10% of neutral)
Dicarboxylic	Glutamic acid, aspartic acid	Carrier-mediated	Rapid
Imino acids and glycine	Proline, hydroxyproline, glycine*	Active, Na$^+$-dependent	Slow

*Shares both the neutral and imino mechanism.
Modified from Gray, G.M., and Cooper, H.L.: Gastroenterology, *61*:535, 1971.

AMINO ACIDS

In contrast to peptide absorption, the transport of free amino acids at the brush border membrane is relatively slow and appears to be the rate-limiting step in the assimilation of that fraction (30 per cent) of dietary protein that is hydrolyzed to amino acids within the intestinal lumen. Intestinal transport of amino acids exhibits specificity for L-stereoisomers, which can be transported against very steep concentration gradients, whereas D-isomers cannot. Amino acids are transported via a carrier-mediated process that is stimulated by sodium and is energy dependent. The energy required for transport of amino acids from lumen to blood is provided by the mechanism that pumps sodium out of the basolateral aspect of the enterocyte, i.e., the Na$^+$-K$^+$ pump. The transport of amino acids out of the cell at the basolateral membrane occurs down a concentration gradient, yet it remains unclear whether this process involves simple diffusion (because of the permeable nature of the basolateral membrane) or a carrier-mediated process.

Four different amino acid transport systems have been described which are based upon carrier affinities for different groups of amino acids (Table 7–4), i.e., (1) neutral, (2) dibasic, (3) dicarboxylic, and (4) imino (and glycine) amino acids. The neutral (monoamino-monocarboxylic) amino acid mechanism transports aliphatic amino acids (e.g., alanine), aromatic amino acids (e.g., tyrosine), and other neutral amino acids (e.g., histidine) at a very rapid rate. Dibasic (diamino) amino acids, such as lysine, are transported by a separate carrier system exhibiting a maximum transport rate which is only one tenth that of the neutral amino acid carrier. This difference may be explained on the basis of the electrical charge of the solute, inasmuch as the dibasic amino acids are transported against an electrical gradient.

The acidic (dicarboxylic) amino acids (e.g., glutamic acid) are also transported by a common carrier. In contrast to the other carrier mechanisms, which transport amino acids against a concentration gradient and require energy, the dicarboxylic amino acid carrier does not require energy, since transport always proceeds along a concentration gradient. The low intracellular concentration of acidic amino acids is explained by the fact that they undergo immediate transamination with pyruvate to yield alanine and a ketoacid. Therefore, alanine appears in portal venous blood during intestinal absorption of dicarboxylic amino acids.

A common carrier mechanism also exists for the transport of imino acids (L-proline and hydroxyproline) and glycine. This transport process proceeds at a very slow rate and may not be physiologically important, because proline and glycine are often absorbed in the form of dipeptides or tripeptides. Glycine shares both the neutral and imino carriers, yet it exhibits a lower affinity for the neutral carrier. Competitive inhibition of amino acid transport occurs at each of the four carriers, for amino acids within and between carrier groups.

Absorption of Native Proteins

Normal adults absorb only minute amounts of undigested protein, because the intestinal mucosa is normally too impermeable for diffusion of macromolecules through the tight junctions and because of the insignificant pinocytotic transport in the enterocytes of adults. Only when the mucosal barrier is disrupted do large quantities of intact proteins gain access to the lamina propria of intestinal villi in adult humans. In some animals (e.g., ruminants), passive immunity is conferred to the suckling neonate by absorption of immunoglobulins contained in colostrum. The absorption of antibodies is accomplished by pinocytosis; the proteins are engulfed by invaginations of the brush border membrane, transferred across the cell, and then released into the interstitial space at the basolateral membrane. This process normally terminates 3 to 18 days after birth. Early feeding of these animals can result in premature "closure" of the mucosal membrane to proteins, suggesting that factors in the colostrum govern the ability of the intestinal enterocyte to transport intact proteins. In humans, this process does not provide significant antibody protection for the newborn; however, there is evidence that infants under three months absorb food antigens more readily than older infants.

Nucleoprotein Digestion and Absorption

Nucleoproteins are normal constituents of ingested animal and plant products which are also hydrolyzed and absorbed in the small intestine. Intraluminal hydrolysis of dietary nucleoproteins is catalyzed by the spectrum of proteolytic enzymes secreted by the pancreas. The endopeptidases and exopeptidases sequentially hydrolyze the histone and protamine components of nucleoproteins to oligopeptides and amino acids, which are ultimately absorbed by the enterocytes. The nucleic acid components (DNA or RNA) are hydrolyzed by the pancreatic enzymes, deoxyribonuclease and ribonuclease, to yield polynucleotides. There are specific phosphodiesterases in the brush border membrane which catalyze the surface hydrolysis of polynucleotides to purine and pyrimidine nucleotides. The nucleotides then undergo surface hydrolysis (catalyzed by nucleotidases) to form nucleosides. There are specific transport mechanisms in the brush border membrane which allow entry of purine and pyrimidine nucleosides into the enterocyte. The capacity of the nucleoside transport pathways is small in comparison to the absorptive capacities for carbohydrates and amino acids; however, the dietary loads are also much smaller.

WATER-SOLUBLE VITAMINS (Table 7–5)

Vitamins are organic substances that are necessary for normal metabolic functions, yet they cannot be manufactured by the body. Therefore, it is essential for these compounds to be absorbed from ingested foods. The water-soluble vitamins generally function as essential cofactors for enzymatic reactions, and they range in size from 176 MW (ascorbic acid) to 1300 MW (cobalamin). A variety of mechanisms, including simple and facilitated diffusion and active transport, is involved in the absorption of water-soluble vitamins. All are absorbed in either the jejunum or ileum. When a carrier molecule is involved in vitamin transport it is located at the brush border membrane, and vitamin transport into the cell is often coupled to sodium. Certain vitamins (e.g., folates and thiamine) are metabolized either while crossing the brush border membrane or within the cytosol. The mechanism(s) by which water-soluble vitamins leave the enterocyte across the basolateral membrane remain unclear; however, it appears that the molecular size and degree of ionization are major factors influencing the mode and rate of exit from the cell. Although all of the water-soluble vitamins have been extensively studied, folic acid and cobalamin (vitamin B_{12}) have received the most attention from gastrointestinal physiologists and gastroenterologists, because blood disorders commonly result from malabsorption of these vitamins.

Folates

Folates are found in a wide variety of foods, including vegetables and nuts. The average American diet provides approximately 0.7 mg of folates per day, while the daily requirement is about 0.1 mg. Seventy to 80 per cent of the dietary folates are polyglutamate conjugates (pteroylpolyglutamates), linked by a γ- rather than the more common α-peptide bond. The remaining dietary folates exist in free form. Gastric and pancreatic enzymes are incapable of cleaving the γ-peptide bond. However, the brush border membrane of enterocytes in the jejunum contains an enzyme (pteroylpolyglutamate hydrolase)

TABLE 7–5. Absorption of Water Soluble Vitamins

Vitamin	Daily Adult Requirement	Site of Absorption	Mechanism of Transport	Major Physiologic Functions
Ascorbic acid (vitamin C)	45 mg	Ileum	Active transport	Maintenance of normal intercellular substances; essential for oxidation reactions
Folic acid	0.1 mg	Jejunum	Facilitated diffusion	Nucleic acid synthesis; promotes growth and maturation of red blood cells
Pyridoxine (vitamin B_6)	2 mg	Jejunum	Simple diffusion	Acts as coenzyme in reactions of amino acid and protein metabolism
Riboflavin (vitamin B_2)	1.8 mg	Jejunum	Facilitated diffusion	Constituent of flavin nucleotide coenzymes
Thiamine (vitamin B_1)	1.5 mg	Jejunum	Active transport	Metabolism of carbohydrates and some amino acids
Cobalamin (vitamin B_{12})	0.003 mg	Ileum	Active transport	Essential for DNA synthesis; promotes growth and maturation of red blood cells
Nicotinamide (niacin)	20 mg	Jejunum	Active transport	Acts as a coenzyme in oxidation reactions

INTESTINAL   EPITHELIAL   MESENTERIC
  LUMEN   CELL   CIRCULATION

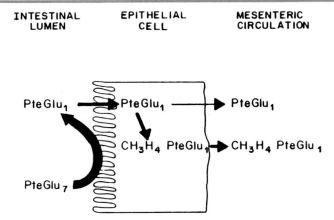

FIGURE 7–20. Digestion and absorption of dietary pteroylpolyglutamates (PteGlu$_7$). Surface hydrolysis of PteGlu$_7$ yields folic acid (PteGlu$_1$), which is transported into the cell. Once in the cell, folic acid either is methylated and reduced (yielding CH$_3$H$_4$PteGlu$_1$) or diffuses into the blood stream. (From Rosenberg, I.H.: Folate absorption and malabsorption. N. Engl. J. Med., 293:1303, 1975.)

which hydrolyzes the polyglutamyl conjugates of folate (Fig. 7–20). Surface hydrolysis of the polyglutamate-folate conjugates (PteGlu$_7$) ultimately yields a monoglutamyl (PteGlu$_1$) product (folic acid) which is transported into the enterocyte by facilitated diffusion. Once within the cell, a large proportion of the folic acid is methylated and reduced to the tetrahydro form (CH$_3$H$_4$PteGlu$_1$). The methylated and nonmethylated forms of folic acid then exit the cell at the basolateral membrane and subsequently bind to folate-binding plasma proteins. Folate malabsorption is a common accompaniment to gastrointestinal disease (e.g., celiac disease) and in patients on a variety of drugs (e.g., sulfasalazine, an agent used to treat ileitis and colitis). Inasmuch as folic acid is essential for red blood cell growth and maturation, folate malabsorption may lead to anemia.

Cobalamin

Cobalamin (vitamin B$_{12}$) is produced by bacteria and enters animal tissues by ingestion of contaminated foods (particularly meat and seafood). The average Western diet contains 5 to 15 μg per day, and the daily adult requirement is 3 μg. Cobalamin is bound to protein (primarily enzymes) in food sources, from which it is liberated by pepsin in the presence of acid. Once cobalamin is liberated from food, it binds with a glycoprotein synthesized by the parietal cells of the stomach called intrinsic factor. One molecule of intrinsic factor tightly binds two molecules of cobalamin. The intrinsic factor-cobalamin complex is delivered to the ileum where it attaches to specific receptors on the brush border membrane (Fig. 7–21). Attachment of the glycoprotein-vitamin complex to the membrane requires calcium and a pH greater than 5.6. Free cobalamin does not bind to the ileal receptor. The translocation of cobalamin into the enterocyte is not understood. It is not known whether intrinsic factor is also taken up by the enterocyte or whether it remains completely on the

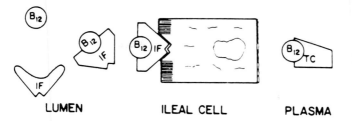

FIGURE 7–21. Sequence of events involved in the intestinal absorption of cyanocobalamin (B_{12}). IF = Intrinsic factor; TC = Transcobalamin. (Modified from Donaldson, R.M. *In* Kramer, M., and Lauterbach, F. (eds.): Intestinal Permeation. Amsterdam, Excerpta Medica, 1977.)

surface of the cell. After extrusion at the basolateral membrane, cobalamin is transported in blood bound to B_{12}-binding globulins called transcobalamins. Cobalamin malabsorption may result from any disorder which depresses intrinsic factor secretion (pernicious anemia), interferes with attachment of the cobalamin-intrinsic factor complex to ileal receptors (severe celiac disease), or impairs uptake into blood (transcobalamin deficiency). Inasmuch as cobalamin is essential for DNA synthesis, cobalamin deficiency significantly impairs the rate of production of rapidly proliferating cells such as erythrocytes.

LIPID DIGESTION AND ABSORPTION

Dietary Lipids

The daily dietary intake of lipids by man in the Western world ranges between 60 and 100 grams. The primary dietary lipids are triglycerides, cholesterol esters, phospholipids, and the fat-soluble vitamins. Triglycerides account for over 90 per cent of dietary lipid. Most of the ingested triglycerides contain long-chain fatty acids (palmitic, stearic, oleic, and linoleic acids) with a smaller proportion (about 10 per cent) containing short- and medium-chain fatty acids (e.g., butyric acid). Dietary triglycerides are derived from animal body and milk fats and from vegetable oils. Lipids, in general, are the most concentrated source of calories in the diet, yielding more than twice as many calories as carbohydrates (9 calories per gram for lipids and 4 calories per gram for carbohydrates). Lipids account for 30 to 40 per cent of the calories in the average diet.

Triglyceride Digestion

Hydrolysis of lipids in the stomach by lingual lipase is limited; therefore, most fat appears in the duodenum in the form ingested. In the alkaline environment of the duodenum, fats are emulsified by fatty acids, monoglycerides, lecithin, and proteins (bile salts contribute relatively little to emulsification). These emulsifying agents act as detergents which physically disperse the fat into minute droplets. Prior to emulsification, fat globules have an average diameter of 1000 Å, which is reduced to 50 Å by emulsification. Emulsification facilitates triglyceride digestion by increasing the total surface area available for the action of pancreatic enzymes, which act only at the surface of the lipid droplets.

The presence of fat (particularly long-chain fatty acids) in the duodenum stimulates the release of cholecystokinin, which, in turn, causes the pancreas to secrete digestive enzymes into the bowel lumen. Among these are the lipolytic enzyme lipase and its cofactor, colipase, both of which play a major role in the hydrolysis of triglycerides. Pancreatic lipase, which is secreted in an active form (rather than a proenzyme), acts only at the oil-water interface but is inactive in the presence of bile salts. Colipase must also be present for lipase to initiate lipid digestion. Unlike lipase, colipase is secreted by the pancreas in the form of a precursor, i.e., procolipase. Procolipase is converted to colipase by trypsin. Colipase recognizes and binds to triglyceride at the oil-water interface, a process requiring the presence of bile salts. One molecule of lipase binds to one molecule of colipase and hydrolysis begins. Therefore, colipase acts as an "anchor" for lipase attachment at the oil-water interface; without colipase, bile salts would not allow lipase to adhere to the surface of fat droplets. Other physiologic advantages of the lipase-colipase interaction are (1) that the optimum pH for lipase action, which is normally 8, is reduced to 6 (near duodenal pH) when colipase binds to lipase and (2) that the inhibition of lipase by bile salts is overcome.

Triglyceride is acted upon by pancreatic lipase to yield two fatty acids (hydrolyzed at the 1 and 3 positions) and a 2-monoglyceride (Fig. 7–22). The lipase sequentially attacks the two outer bonds of the triglyceride molecule, producing, at first, a diglyceride and one fatty acid, then two fatty acids and a monoglyceride. The monoglyceride can be converted into glycerol and a fatty acid by pancreatic lipase. However, the latter reaction requires shifting of the ester bond to the 1 position. This isomerization proceeds at a slower rate than the absorption of 2-monoglycerides by the enterocyte.

Pancreatic lipase also exhibits substrate specificity, i.e., the rate of hydrolysis of triglycerides with butyric or propionic acid chains is 2.5 times that observed for triglycerides with long-chain fatty acids. The rate of triglyceride hydrolysis by lipase is extremely rapid, owing to the large excess of enzyme secreted by the pancreas in response to a meal. It has been estimated (based on the amount of lipase in intestinal contents) that humans have the capacity to digest 140 grams of fat per minute. Since daily fat ingestion rarely exceeds 150 grams, there is over a thousandfold excess of lipase in the intestinal lumen. Up to 80 per cent of the total fatty acids present in triglyceride are liberated by the time the fat has reached the middle of the duodenum.

Human milk contains a nonspecific lipase that is activated by bile salts and is resistant to gastric acid. The enzyme has been shown to assist in the digestion of fat in infants. Cow's milk does not possess this lipase. Although milk lipase

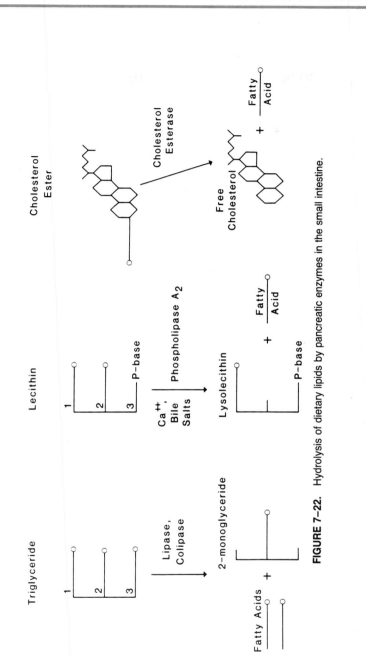

FIGURE 7–22. Hydrolysis of dietary lipids by pancreatic enzymes in the small intestine.

may contribute to triglyceride digestion in the small bowel, it is clear that this enzyme is not essential for the assimilation of dietary fat.

Phospholipid Digestion

Dietary phospholipids (e.g., lecithin) are hydrolyzed in the intestinal lumen by the pancreatic enzyme phospholipase A_2. The phospholipase is secreted in pancreatic juice as an inactive proenzyme (prophospholipase A_2), which is activated in the lumen by trypsin. In the presence of calcium and bile salts, phospholipase A_2 hydrolyzes lecithin at the fatty acid ester bond at position 2 to yield lysolecithin and a fatty acid (Fig. 7–22). Phosphatidylethanolamine and phosphatidylserine are also substrates for phospholipase A_2.

Cholesterol Digestion

Cholesterol is found in the human diet principally in the form of esters. Intestinal hydrolysis of cholesterol esters to cholesterol and free fatty acids is catalyzed by the enzyme cholesterol esterase (Fig. 7–22). This enzyme is present in pancreatic juice and acts primarily on unsaturated fatty acids. Intraluminal hydrolysis of cholesterol esters is of importance, since cholesterol is absorbed as free cholesterol rather than in the ester form. Cholesterol esterases also occur inside the epithelial cells of the small intestine, where they appear to play a role in the re-esterification of cholesterol.

Solubilization of Lipid Digestion Products

Before the products of lipid digestion can be absorbed by the intestine, they must be solubilized in the aqueous phase of the lumen contents. This absorption is achieved by incorporating the lipolytic products into bile salt micelles. At the concentrations found in bile and the intestinal lumen, bile salts form cylindrical aggregates (micelles) in which the hydrophilic portion of the molecule faces the aqueous phase of the solution while the hydrophobic portion faces inward, away from the aqueous phase. Lipids such as cholesterol, lysolecithin, monoglycerides, and free fatty acids (particularly long-chain) enter the lipid-soluble interior of the bile salt micelle, forming larger mixed micelles. Micellar solubilization increases the concentration of lipolytic products in the aqueous phase by a factor of 1000. Although the micelle (70 to 400 Å, diameter) is much larger than a fatty acid molecule, it increases the rate of delivery of fatty acids to the enterocytes by 100 to 200 times owing to the ability of the particle to traverse the unstirred water layer adjacent to the brush border. Micellar solubilization of monoglycerides and fatty acids removes them from the oil-water interface at which pancreatic lipase acts, thereby enhancing digestion of the remaining triglyceride.

Cellular Uptake of Lipolytic Products

Mixed micelles formed in the intestinal lumen must interact with three diffusion barriers before the lipid contents can enter the enterocyte: (1) the unstirred water layer overlying the enterocyte, (2) the mucous coat covering the brush border membrane, and (3) the lipid bilayer membrane that makes up the brush border. Both the unstirred water layer and mucous coat significantly reduce the movement of micelles (and long-chain fatty acids) relative to free diffusion in water. Although the micelle per se does not permeate the lipid bilayer membrane, its lipid constituents (monoglycerides, fatty acids, cholesterol, lysolecithin) dissolve into the lipid bilayer membrane of the cell and thus enter it by passive nonionic diffusion. The rate of exchange of lipolytic products between the micelles and lipid membrane of the cell is very rapid and is primarily determined by the solubility of the lipolytic product in the cell membrane and its concentration gradient across the membrane. Therefore, in the overall process of diffusional micellar transport of lipid from the intestinal lumen to within the enterocyte, the static water layer and mucous coat are the more significant barriers. Once the lipid contents of the micelle enter the intestinal cell, the emptied bile salt micelle picks up another load of lipid hydrolysis products for delivery to the enterocyte.

While long-chain fatty acids and cholesterol must be incorporated into bile salt micelles before absorption, solubilization in micelles is not a requirement for the absorption of short- (C2 to C4) and medium- (C6 to C10) chain fatty acids. Short- and medium-chain fatty acids and the triglycerides of those acids are sufficiently water soluble that they can reach the enterocyte by simple diffusion; i.e., passage through the unstirred water layer and mucous coat is not the rate-limiting step in their absorption. This is demonstrated by the fact that approximately 30 per cent of an oral dose of medium-chain triglyceride is absorbed intact. Nonetheless, a proportion of the medium-chain fatty acids in the intestinal lumen is incorporated into micelles and is transported to the enterocyte membrane in the same manner as long-chain fatty acids.

Intracellular Metabolism of Lipid Digestion Products

MONOGLYCERIDES AND FATTY ACIDS

After monoglycerides and fatty acids diffuse through the bilipid layer and enter the cell, they are transferred to the microsomes of the endoplasmic reticulum for resynthesis into triglycerides (Fig. 7–23). Transfer of long-chain fatty acids to the microsomes is facilitated by a transport protein (fatty acid–binding protein) which solubilizes the lipid i the polar interior of the enterocyte. (A protein that transports monoglycerides has not been discovered.) The endoplasmic reticulum contains all of the enzymes and cofactors necessary for re-esterification of fatty acids and monoglycerides into triglycerides. Two metabolic pathways are involved in the synthesis of triglycerides in enterocytes:

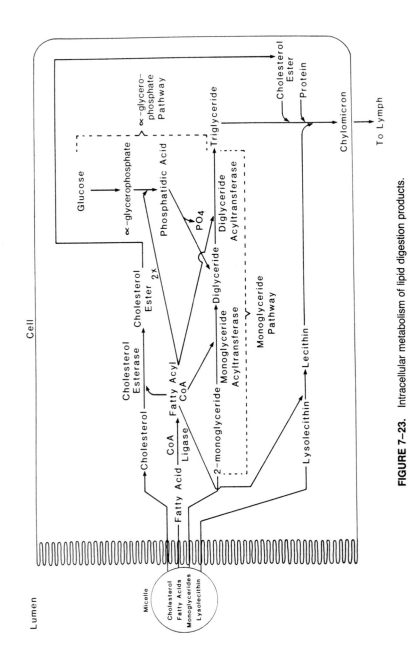

FIGURE 7–23. Intracellular metabolism of lipid digestion products.

the monoglyceride acylation pathway and the α-glycerophosphate pathway. Both pathways utilize absorbed fatty acids with chain lengths greater than twelve carbons; smaller fatty acids are not re-esterified into triglyceride but diffuse directly into portal blood. The monoglyceride acylation pathway is the most important route for triglyceride resynthesis. This involves the activation of absorbed fatty acids by the enzyme fatty acid CoA ligase and subsequent attachment of the activated fatty acid to a monoglyceride, a reaction catalyzed by the enzyme monoglyceride acyltransferase. The third fatty acid is added by diglyceride acyltransferase to complete the resynthesis of triglyceride. In addition to the monoglyceride acylation pathway, the enterocyte can produce triglyceride by esterification of absorbed fatty acid with glycerol phosphate derived from intracellular metabolism of glucose. The phosphatidic acid (glycerol phosphate–fatty acid ester) is dephosphorylated and then esterified with an additional fatty acid to produce a triglyceride. The phosphatidic acid pathway normally plays a minor role in intestinal triglyceride formation.

CHOLESTEROL

Cholesterol is almost insoluble in water and therefore enters the intestinal cell less readily than long-chain fatty acids and monoglycerides. Only half of the luminal cholesterol enters the mucosal cell. Once within the cell, dietary cholesterol is re-esterified mainly with oleic acid, a reaction catalyzed by cholesterol esterase (Fig. 7–23). The enterocytes of the ileum are a major site of cholesterol synthesis in the body. The cholesterol biosynthetic pathway in the ileum is the same as that described for liver. Because of its capacity for absorbing dietary cholesterol and its ability to synthesize cholesterol, the small intestine plays an important role in the regulation of body cholesterol levels.

PHOSPHOLIPIDS

The products of pancreatic enzyme digestion of phospholipids are fatty acids and lysolecithin; the latter is less efficiently absorbed by the enterocytes. Once inside the absorptive cell (Fig. 7–23), nonesterified phospholipids such as lysolecithin are acylated by microsomal enzymes to form esters (e.g., lecithin). The rate of re-esterification of phospholipid is related to its need in the assembly and transport of chylomicrons. Other phospholipids (e.g., sphingolipids) are degraded in the enterocyte. Phospholipid is essential for normal structure and function of membranes such as the brush border membrane. A large fraction of absorbed phospholipid exits the cell in chylomicrons; however, some of the dietary phospholipid is incorporated into the cellular membranes of the enterocyte.

Chylomicron Formation and Transport

As fat absorption proceeds, droplets of resynthesized triglycerides (and some cholesterol) fill the rough endoplasmic reticulum. The triglyceride droplets then migrate to the smooth endoplasmic reticulum, where newly synthe-sized phospholipid is added to the lipid droplet. The prechylomicron is then transported to the Golgi apparatus where a glycoprotein coat is added. The chylomicrons are then packaged into secretory vesicles, which fuse with the lateral portions of the cell membrane. The nascent chylomicrons are subse-quently released from the secretory vesicles into the lateral intercellular spaces. The entire process of chylomicron formation and release, from cell uptake of fat to release into the lateral intercellular spaces, requires only 12 to 15 minutes. The chylomicrons must then pass through the basement membrane, traverse the lamina propria, and finally accumulate in the lymph of the terminal lacteals, to which chylomicrons impart a milky appearance. The chylomicrons ultimately gain access to the blood stream via the thoracic duct, which empties into the subclavian vein.

Chylomicrons are large particles ranging in size between 750 and 6000 Å. The variable size of chylomicrons appears to be related to the rates of fatty acid absorption and triglyceride resynthesis. Their chemical composition is approx-imately 90 per cent triglyceride, 7 per cent phospholipid, 2 per cent cholesterol, and 1 per cent protein. The inner core of the chylomicron contains almost all the triglyceride and most of the cholesterol. Phospholipid covers 80 to 90 per cent, while protein covers 10 to 20 per cent of the chylomicron surface.

The intestinal cell also forms small lipoprotein particles called very low density lipoproteins (VLDL), which appear to be a major route of transport of dietary cholesterol into blood. The VLDL contain more cholesterol and protein, yet less triglyceride, than chylomicrons. The processes of VLDL formation and release are much like those described above for chylomicrons. Studies in an-imals indicate that VLDL particles are primarily responsible for transporting endogenous lipids from enterocytes to lymph in the fasting state.

The partition of absorbed fatty acids between portal venous blood and intestinal lymph is largely determined by the chain length of the fatty acid. Long-chain fatty acids ($> 14C$) are transported mainly as resynthesized tri-glyceride in the chylomicrons and VLDL of lymph. The lipoproteins (VLDL, chylomicrons) cannot gain access to the blood circulation via intestinal capillaries because the fenestral openings in the capillary endothelium (500 Å diameter) are too small to allow permeation by the lipid particles. As much as 20 per cent of the long-chain fatty acids absorbed by the small bowel enter the portal vein bound to plasma proteins such as albumin. Fatty acids of intermediate chain length (10 to 14C) are removed from the intestine both in chylomicrons and by diffusion into blood. Because short-chain fatty acids ($< 8C$) are water soluble, they readily diffuse from the enterocyte into blood capillaries, which is their primary route of transport out of the intestine.

Absorption of Fat-Soluble Vitamins

The fat-soluble vitamins (A, D, E, and K) are absorbed primarily in the proximal small intestine by mechanism(s) which require bile salts. They are all relatively nonpolar molecules and must be incorporated into micelles for efficient absorption. After entry into the mucosal cell, the fat-soluble vitamins become associated with chylomicrons, VLDL, or both, from which they gain access to the blood circulation via lymph.

Vitamin A (retinol) is derived only from animal sources, but plant carotenoids such as β-carotene can be converted in vivo to retinol. Retinol is required for the formation of visual (retinol) pigments, and it is necessary for the normal growth and proliferation of epithelial cells. It is absorbed in the small intestine by a carrier-mediated process. Once retinol enters the enterocyte it is esterified to fatty acids and subsequently incorporated into chylomicrons. The provitamin, β-carotene, is split by an intracellular enzyme (dioxygenase) to yield two molecules of retinaldehyde, which are subsequently reduced to retinol.

Vitamin D is produced endogenously; however, significant quantities of both vitamins D_2 (ergocalciferol) and D_3 (cholecalciferol) are absorbed in the small intestine. Vitamin D_3 occurs naturally in high concentrations in fish liver oils, and vitamins D_2 and D_3 are added to fortify certain foods. Absorption takes place via a passive process which occurs in both the proximal and distal intestine. Vitamin D plays an important role in the regulation of plasma calcium levels; a major effect of the vitamin is stimulation of intestinal calcium absorption (see Fig. 7–9).

Vitamin E actually represents a group of lipid-soluble derivatives with varying biologic potency; the most active of these compounds is α-tocopherol. The richest sources of vitamin E in the diet are seed oils and wheat germ oil. A major physiologic function of α-tocopherol is to prevent the oxidation of unsaturated fatty acids in cellular membranes. Intestinal absorption of vitamin E requires both pancreatic juice and bile. Pancreatic enzymes facilitate vitamin E absorption by hydrolyzing esters of the vitamin and by providing lipolytic products for enhanced solubilization of the vitamin. Once in the mucosal cell, vitamin E is incorporated into chylomicrons.

Vitamin K represents a group of compounds that are required for the synthesis of clotting factors produced by the liver. Dietary vitamin K is found principally in green vegetables. The naturally occurring K vitamins are insoluble in water; however, synthetic forms of the vitamin such as menadione, which lack the long hydrocarbon chain, are somewhat water-soluble. As a result of the different solubility characteristics, the naturally occurring and synthetic forms are absorbed by different mechanisms. An energy-requiring, saturable transport mechanism is involved in the absorption of naturally occurring forms, while the synthetic form is absorbed by a passive process. Once within the mucosal cell, the naturally occurring forms are incorporated into chylomicrons and then transferred to the lymphatics. By contrast, the synthetic form of vitamin K is removed from the intestine by the portal venous route.

MOTILITY

Coordinated contractions of the external muscle layers of the small bowel optimize the processes of digestion and absorption by (1) mixing the chyme

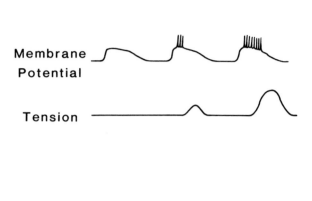

Membrane
Potential

Tension

FIGURE 7–24. Relationship between slow waves, spike activity, and generation of tension in intestinal smooth muscle. Note that smooth muscle contraction (increased tension) occurs only when spike potentials are present on the slow waves. The number of spike potentials is directly related to the strength of the contraction. (Modified from Cohen, S., and Snape, W.J., Jr.: Movement of the small and large intestine. *In* Sleisenger, M.H., and Fordtran, J.S. (eds.): Gastrointestinal Disease: Pathophysiology, Diagnosis, Management. Philadelphia, W.B. Saunders, 1983, p. 859.)

with digestive secretions, (2) repeatedly exposing the lumen contents to the digestive and absorptive surface of the mucosa, and (3) moving the chyme down the intestine. The inner circular muscle layer is considered to play a more important role in the mixing and propulsion of chyme. Intestinal motility represents a coordinated series of contractions which serve to assure the slow passage of chyme through the bowel so that the residue of one meal leaves the ileum as another meal is being ingested. This coordination of motor activity is the result of intrinsic properties of smooth muscle cells, as well as nervous (local plexuses and extrinsic) and humoral (endocrine or paracrine) influences.

Intrinsic Properties of Smooth Muscle Cells

As in the stomach, the contractions of the small intestine are ultimately governed by the basal electrical rhythm (slow waves) of the smooth muscle cells. The slow waves per se do not evoke muscular contractions; instead, they govern the rate at which spike activity can occur. Spike potentials, which occur only during the depolarization phase of the slow waves, lead to contraction of the muscle. The strength of contraction is directly proportional to the frequency of the spike potentials. The relationships between slow waves, spike potentials, and muscle contractions are illustrated in Figure 7–24.

The frequency and temporal distribution of slow waves are not the same in all regions of the small bowel. In the duodenum, the frequency of the slow waves is 12 cycles per minute, while in the distal ileum it is only 9 cycles per minute. If the entire small intestine is divided into a series of short segments, each segment will have its own characteristic frequency of slow waves, with a gradual, linear decline in intrinsic frequency from proximal duodenum to distal ileum. However, in the intact intestine this decline in slow wave frequency is not a simple linear process. It is a gradual stepwise decline, consisting of a series of frequency plateaus (Fig. 7–25). The 12 cycles per minute frequency

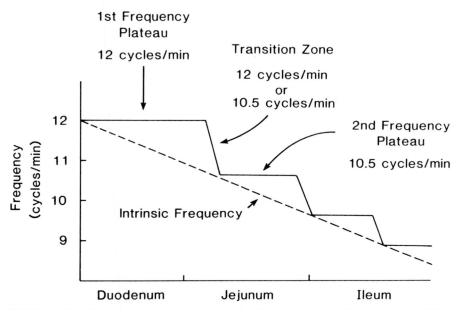

FIGURE 7–25. The frequency of slow waves along the small intestine. The stepwise solid line shows the frequency along the intact gut, 12/min in the duodenum and upper jejunum and declining to 9/min in the ileum. The lower dashed line represents the intrinsic frequency displayed by short, isolated segments of the intestine.

found in the duodenum extends up to 10 cm into the jejunum, after which it declines to a lower frequency, where it remains steady along another given length of gut and then declines further, and so on, until the lowest frequency (9 cycles per minute) is achieved in the ileum. Each frequency plateau is separated by a short segment of bowel whose frequency shifts between that of the upper and lower segment.

The existence of slow wave frequency plateaus along the small intestine can be explained in terms of pacemaker oscillators that have high intrinsic frequencies. The pacemaker oscillators dominate over adjacent coupled oscillators of lower intrinsic frequencies. In the upper duodenum, smooth muscle cells with a high intrinsic slow wave frequency serve as pacemaker oscillators that impose their frequency on adjacent smooth muscle cells having a lower intrinsic frequency via cell-to-cell electrical coupling. Thus, along the duodenum and the proximal jejunum the smooth muscle cells have the same slow wave frequency until a point is reached where the intrinsic frequency is too low to be influenced by the higher pacemaker frequency. The smooth muscle cells in this portion of the gut then assume the role of pacemaker oscillators which dominate aborally located cells, thereby establishing another lower frequency plateau. The transition zone between adjacent frequency plateaus is

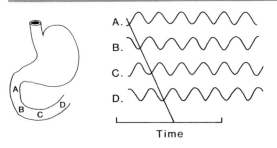

A.

B.

C.

D.

Time

FIGURE 7–26. Slow waves along different points on a frequency plateau in the upper small intestine. A line is drawn through corresponding slow-wave cycles from each point, illustrating the proximal to distal phase lag of the slow waves.

characterized by a frequency which shifts between that of the higher and lower plateau values.

The aboral gradient in the frequency plateaus ensures that chyme moves from a region of higher potential contractile frequency to a region of lower potential frequency. However, the question arises as to how chyme moves along a given frequency plateau, where the frequency of slow waves is the same. The answer lies in the observation that the slow waves along a frequency plateau do not occur simultaneously at all loci, i.e., there is an aborally oriented phase lag. This phase lag is created by the time required for the propagation of the pacemaker frequency (Fig. 7–26). Table 7–6 lists some of the factors which influence slow wave frequency in the small intestine.

Nervous Control of Motility

Both intrinsic and extrinsic nerves influence the contractile activity of the smooth muscle cells of the muscularis externa of the small bowel. The intrinsic nerves are primarily confined to the myenteric and submucosal plexuses. Because of its strategic location between the circular and longitudinal muscle layers, the myenteric plexus is more important in regulating intestinal contractions. Contractions of both longitudinal and circular muscle layers are

TABLE 7–6.   Factors Influencing Slow Wave Frequency in the Small Intestine

Factors Increasing Slow Wave Frequency
pyrexia
hyperthyroidism

Factors Decreasing Slow Wave Frequency
duodenal compression or transection*
hypothermia
hypothyroidism
hypoglycemia
malabsorption syndromes

Factors Not Altering Slow Wave Frequency
cholinergic compounds
topical anesthetics
extrinsic nerve stimulation
ingestion of food

*The slow wave frequency proximal to the affected area is not altered.

brought about by neuronal release of acetylcholine. Since the longitudinal muscle layer contains at least ten times more muscarinic cholinergic receptors than the circular muscle layer, it is far more sensitive to locally released acetylcholine. Indeed, longitudinal muscle contraction may be exclusively mediated by acetylcholine. The most notable influence of the neurons of the myenteric plexus on the circular muscle layer is one of tonic inhibition. The inhibitory neurons are continuously active in all nonsphincteric regions of the gut where they suppress contractions of circular smooth muscle. The neurotransmitter involved is believed to be either a purine nucleotide or vasoactive intestinal polypeptide. Momentary decrements in the discharge frequency of these neurons would result in an increased spike activity and subsequent contraction of the gut. The presence of both excitatory and inhibitory neurons allows for integrated control of intestinal contractions and is of primary importance in initiating the patterns of motility observed in the gut (see below).

Extrinsic neural control of motility is achieved via parasympathetic and sympathetic inputs to the myenteric plexus. The vagus nerve contains two populations of preganglionic parasympathetic fibers, one synapsing with the cholinergic excitatory neurons, the other synapsing with the inhibitory neurons. Although vagal stimulation generally elicits contractions of the intestine, suppression of ongoing spontaneous contractions has also been observed.

The sympathetic supply to the intestinal musculature is derived from preganglionic axons leaving the spinal cord (at T-9 to T-10) and synapsing in the celiac and superior mesenteric ganglia (see Fig. 1–6). The postganglionic fibers issuing from the celiac ganglia innervate the upper duodenum, whereas those leaving the superior mesenteric ganglia innervate the remainder of the small bowel. The adrenergic fibers from both ganglia synapse primarily on neurons within the myenteric plexus, although a few do terminate on smooth muscle cells. Sympathetic activation consistently results in inhibition of intestinal contractions at nonsphincteric sites, either by preventing the release of acetylcholine from intramural neurons or by activating adrenergic receptors on the smooth muscle cells.

The involvement of extrinsic autonomic nerves in the motility patterns observed in the fed or fasted states is minimal. However, the extrinsic nerves are important in modifying motor activity via reflex arcs originating either in the gastrointestinal tract or elsewhere.

Humoral Factors Controlling Motility

The smooth muscle cells of the intestinal wall are sensitive to a variety of circulating substances. Table 7–7 lists the substances produced within the gastrointestinal tract that influence motor activity of the small intestine. Some of the compounds are neurotransmitters or neurocrines, while others are endocrines or paracrines. Some have a more ubiquitous distribution, being localized to both endocrine cells and nerve terminals. Although all of the chemicals listed in Table 7–7 can alter the contractile activity of the small intestine under

TABLE 7–7.   Various Substances of Gastrointestinal Origin Altering Intestinal Motility

Agents Increasing Motility	Agents Decreasing Motility
Acetylcholine*	Norepinephrine*
Serotonin (5-HT)*†	Somatostatin*†
Gastrin†	Secretin†
Cholecystokinin†	Vasoactive Intestinal Peptide (VIP)*†
Enkephalin†	Enteroglucagon†
Motilin†	Gastric Inhibitory Polypeptide†
Substance P*†	Purines*

*Found in nerve terminals of the myenteric plexus.
†Found in mucosal endocrine cells.

experimental conditions, not all of them have been shown to play a physiologic role in the regulation of intestinal motility.

Patterns of Intestinal Muscle Contraction

INTERDIGESTIVE PATTERN

During the interdigestive period, a characteristic sequence of motor activity occurs at regular intervals. The contractile activity originates in the upper duodenum (or gastric antrum) and sweeps down the length of the small bowel. This *migrating motility complex* (MMC) has been divided into three phases (Fig. 7–27): a period of no activity (Phase I), a period of random activity (Phase II), followed by a period of intense contractile activity (Phase III). The intense contractile activity during Phase III is associated with aboral propulsion of lumen contents. The function of the MMC is considered to be that of a "housekeeper" which prevents bacterial overgrowth of the small intestine during fasting.

The migrating motility complexes occur approximately every 140 to 150 minutes; the speed of migration is coordinated so that as one complex terminates in the ileum, another is beginning in the upper gut. In addition, there is a gradient in the velocity of migration along the small intestine, the velocity being greater in the duodenum than in the ileum. This gradient in velocity of the motor complex is attributed to the gradient of slow wave frequency along the gut.

Humoral factors are primarily responsible for the initiation of migrating motility complexes. The peptide motilin, found mainly in the mucosa of the proximal intestine, is considered to be the humoral mediator. Circulating levels of motilin rise during Phase III of the MMC. Furthermore, exogenously administered motilin induces premature initiation of MMC's in the duodenum that migrate to the ileum. The role of extrinsic nerves in modulating the MMC appears minimal, while the role of the myenteric plexus remains unclear.

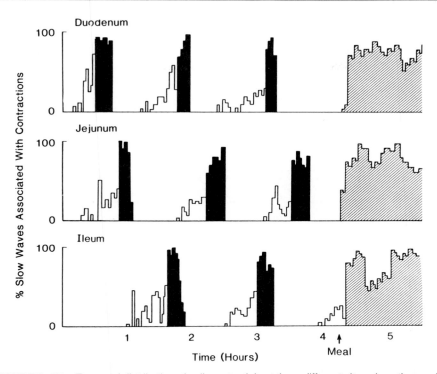

FIGURE 7–27. Temporal distribution of spike potentials at three different sites along the small intestine in the interdigestive period. Periods of no spike potentials correspond to Phase 1 (solid line), periods of 10 to 50 per cent activity correspond to Phase 2 (clear bars), and periods of 90 to 100 per cent activity correspond to Phase III (solid bars) of the MMC. Note how the complexes recur at each site and how each phase of the complex appears to migrate aborally. Note, also, that the pattern of spike activity is changed after ingestion of a meal (at arrow). (Modified from Weisbrodt, N.W.: Motility of the small intestine. *In* Johnson, L.R. (ed.): Physiology of the Gastrointestinal Tract, Vol. 1. New York, Raven Press, 1981, p. 420.)

DIGESTIVE PATTERN

Feeding interrupts the migrating motility complex and initiates a different pattern of intestinal contractions. Unlike the discrete phases of the MMC, the fed pattern is characterized by random motor activity (groups of 1 to 3 sequential contractions) with much shorter intervals of inactivity (5 to 40 seconds). The exact number of contractions per unit time is dictated by the slow waves and depends on the physical and chemical composition of the food ingested. Twice as many contractions occur when solid food is ingested than when an equicaloric amount of liquid is consumed. In addition, the three major classes of foodstuffs have different effects on contractile activity, with carbohydrates stimulating the largest number of bursts, followed by proteins and lipids. The muscle contractions that occur during the fed state have been classified into two types: segmental and peristaltic.

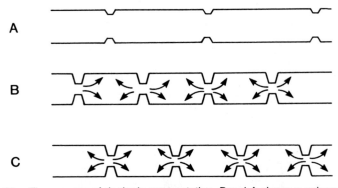

FIGURE 7–28.   The process of rhythmic segmentation. Panel A shows a quiescent gut, and panels B and C illustrate the sequence of contractions that move intestinal contents to and fro.

Segmentation

Rhythmic segmental contractions represent the most frequent type of motor activity occurring after meals. Segmentation consists of cyclic contractions and relaxations of the circular muscle layer at any given site along the gut (Fig. 7–28). Initially, a small segment of bowel (< 2 cm in length) contracts while adjacent segments are relaxed. Subsequently, the contracted segment relaxes while the previously relaxed adjacent segments contract. At any given site along the small bowel, the rate of segmental contractions is either equal to or some multiple of the intrinsic slow wave frequency. Although the basal electrical rhythm determines the maximal number of segmental contractions, neural input from the myenteric plexus plays an important role in coordinating the contraction-relaxation cycles of adjacent segments. Removal of the tonic inhibitory input to a narrow band of circular muscle results in local contraction that does not spread, within the syncytium, to adjacent segments, since the latter are still under the influence of the inhibitory neurons. Contractile activity of the longitudinal muscle does not contribute significantly to the segmental pattern of contractions.

Segmental contractions of the small intestine serve to mix the chyme by continuously displacing it to and fro within the lumen. They also tend to move chyme in an aboral direction. The underlying basis for aboral transport is the relationship between slow waves and segmentation. Because of the proximal-to-distal phase lag of the slow waves on a frequency plateau, individual contractions tend to follow contractions in more proximal segments; the net result is an aboral propulsion of chyme along a given frequency plateau. The aborally declining frequency gradient along the entire small bowel also provides a mechanism for downward movement of chyme. Contractions of the bowel wall not

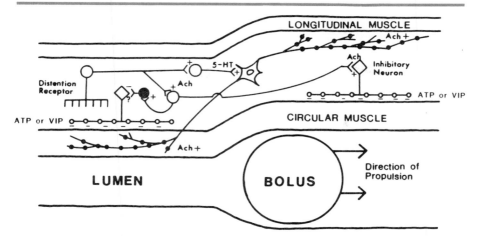

FIGURE 7–29. Schematic diagram of the neural circuitry controlling intestinal circular and longitudinal muscles during the peristaltic reflex, which results in a muscular contraction upstream and relaxation downstream to the bolus. In response to distention of the gut by the bolus, the longitudinal muscle downstream contracts (activation of excitatory cholinergic nerves) and the circular muscle relaxes (increased activity of the inhibitory, purinergic, or peptidergic nerves). Upstream to the bolus the circular muscle contracts (decreased activity of the inhibitory, purinergic, or peptidergic neurons coupled with activation of excitatory cholinergic nerves). (Adapted from Wood, J.D.: Physiology of the enteric nervous system. *In* Johnson, L.R. (ed.): Physiology of the Gastrointestinal Tract, Vol. 1. New York, Raven Press, 1981, p. 32.)

only generate a pressure for propulsion of chyme but also impose a resistance to the movement of chyme. It is generally held, however, that intestinal contractions contribute more to an increase in resistance than propulsion of chyme. Since segmental contractions are less frequent aborally than orally, the average resistance is lower in the ileum than the duodenum. Thus, chyme gradually moves toward the ileum.

Peristaltic Contractions

Peristaltic contractions occur much less frequently than segmental contractions. These contractile waves move chyme aborally for a few centimeters and therefore involve coordinated sequential contractions of both circular and longitudinal muscle layers (Fig. 7–29). The peristaltic wave, sometimes referred to as the peristaltic reflex, consists of a wave of contraction coupled to a downstream wave of relaxation. Distention of the intestinal lumen by a bolus of chyme initiates the reflex via the nerves of the myenteric plexus. Coordinated neuronal activity elicits contraction of longitudinal muscle and a concomitant relaxation of circular muscle immediately "downstream" from the bolus. This contraction and concomitant relaxation serves to increase the radius of the lumen and thereby reduce the resistance to the movement of chyme. The contraction of longitudinal muscle is a result of neuronal release of acetylcholine, while the relaxation of circular muscle is due to increased discharge of the inhibitory neurons. Behind the bolus, the circular muscle contracts and longitudinal muscle relaxes; the net effect is an increase in lumen pressure which propels the bolus into the dilated portion. The "upstream" contraction of circular muscle results from a reduction in the activity of the inhibitory neurons as well as the activation of cholinergic neurons. Relaxation of the longitudinal muscle results from a decreased discharge of cholinergic neurons to this muscle or is simply a passive response to circular muscle contraction.

The polarity of the peristaltic reflex is programmed by the neuronal circuitry of the myenteric plexus. Placement of a bolus of material in the lumen of the small intestine generally results in contraction oral to the bolus and relaxation aboral to the bolus. However, retroperistalsis, or a reversal of the polarity of the reflex, can occur, and chyme can be moved in the oral direction. Retroperistalsis is rare and usually occurs under abnormal circumstances such as vomiting or excess distention of the bowel.

Other Contractile Activity

Contents of the lumen can be mixed by contractions of specialized portions of the mucosa as well as by contractions of the muscularis externa. The muscularis mucosae and the villi both contain smooth muscles which contract spontaneously. Contractions of the muscularis mucosae alter the pattern of folds and ridges of the mucosa (plicae circulares). The contractile activity of the muscularis mucosae increases after a meal, which serves to mix the chyme and expose it to different areas of the mucosal epithelium. The villi of the intestinal mucosa can contract and thereby shorten. Individual villi contract at irregular intervals. The frequency of villus contractions is highest in the duodenum and decreases progressively toward the ileum, where villi seldom contract. The frequency of villus contractions increases after meals, which aids in stirring or mixing the unstirred water layer immediately adjacent to the mucosal epithelium, thereby decreasing the resistance which this barrier offers to absorption of various nutrients (particularly lipids). Villikinin, a hormone produced by the intestinal mucosa, may mediate the postprandial villus contractions. Contractions of the villi also aid in emptying the central lacteals and facilitate the flow of lymph.

Initiation of the Digestive Contraction Pattern

The mixing and propulsive contractions of the postprandial period are initiated by several factors which are brought into play by the ingestion of food. The presence of chyme in the intestinal lumen initiates contractions characteristic of the fed state, a response mediated by the neurons of the myenteric plexus or locally released chemicals (paracrines or neurocrines) or both. However, chyme in the lumen is not a prerequisite for disruption of the interdigestive contractile pattern (MMC) and appearance of the fed pattern. A shift to postprandial contractile activity is also observed in segments of the bowel which are denied contact with chyme. Therefore, extrinsic influences (nerves or hormones) must also be involved. Parasympathetic nerves play a minor role, since vagotomy does not appreciably affect the shift in motility induced by feeding. The role of the sympathetic nerves has not been assessed, but their general inhibitory effects on gut motility suggest that they are not involved. The gastrointestinal hormones are the most likely "extrinsic" factors responsible for the postprandial contractile activity. Exogenous administration of gastrin and cholecystokinin to fasted animals can inhibit the MMC and initiate contractions similar to those observed after feeding. It is quite probable that a complex interaction of factors operating locally and at distant sites along the bowel is responsible for disruption of the MMC and initiation of the digestive pattern of contractions.

Duration of the Digestive Contraction Pattern

Segmental and peristaltic contractions are present for three to four hours after the ingestion of food. The exact duration of the interruption of the MMC by feeding is dependent on the amount and chemical composition of the ingested food. There is a direct linear correlation between the amount of food ingested and the duration of the digestive pattern of contractions. The type of nutrients present in the food also affect the digestive phase, i.e., lipids having a greater effect than sugars, and sugars a greater effect than proteins in prolonging the digestive contractions.

Transit Time of Chyme

The transit of chyme through the small bowel after a meal is slow enough to allow for adequate digestion and absorption of nutrients. The rate of aboral transit is not uniform but is dependent on the relative frequency of segmental and peristaltic contractions. At any given time, chyme may be either moving to and fro as a result of segmental contractions or be moving rapidly for a few centimeters by peristaltic waves. In general, however, chyme moves aborally at a rate of 1 to 4 cm per minute, the velocity of transit being more rapid in the duodenum than in the ileum.

The Ileocecal Junction

As chyme moves gradually down the intestine most of the nutrients, electrolytes, and water are absorbed, leaving only a small volume of residue to pass into the colon (approximately 1.5 liters per day). The flow of chyme between the small intestine and colon is regulated by a 4-cm segment of the terminal ileum, called the ileocecal junction (Fig. 7–30). This structure has two anatomically distinct features that allow it to control the flow of chyme: a sphincter and a valve. The last few centimeters of the ileum are characterized by a thickened muscular (circular) coat that is referred to as the ileocecal sphincter. This sphincter is tonically constricted and generates an intraluminal pressure of about 20 mm Hg. The ability of the sphincter to remain contracted is attributed to the intrinsic properties of its smooth muscle cells. However, intrinsic

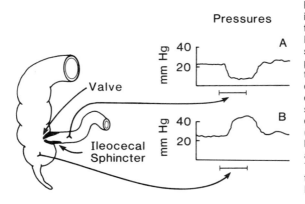

FIGURE 7–30. Response of the ileocecal sphincter to distention of the ileum (*A*) and cecum (*B*). *A*, Distention of the ileum causes the sphincter to relax and the drop in pressure allows chyme to flow into the colon. *B*, Distention of the cecum causes the sphincter to contract and the increase in pressure helps prevent the reflux of cecal contents into the ileum. (Modified from Guyton, A.C.: Textbook of Medical Physiology. Philadelphia, W.B. Saunders, 1981, p. 797; and Johnson, L.R.: Gastrointestinal Physiology, 2nd ed. St. Louis, C.V. Mosby, 1981, p. 40.)

and extrinsic nerves modulate the tone of the sphincter. Distention of the terminal ileum relaxes the sphincter, while distention of the cecum causes it to contract (Fig. 7–30); both responses are mediated by reflex arcs in the myenteric plexus.

Both branches of the autonomic nervous system have a stimulatory effect on the ileocecal junction. Stimulation of either the vagus (parasympathetic) or splanchnic and lumbar (sympathetic) nerves causes a cholinergic-mediated constriction of the ileocecal sphincter. Another feature of the ileocecal junction is the valve formed by the portion of the terminal ileum which protrudes into the cecum. This valve shuts in response to high cecal pressures and can oppose a pressure head of up to 40 mm Hg.

The zone of high pressure generated by the ileocecal sphincter offers resistance to the emptying of chyme into the colon, thereby allowing more time for absorption. As chyme progressively accumulates in and distends the distal ileum, reflex relaxation of the sphincter occurs, and chyme passes into the colon. If colonic contents are not moved analward but accumulate and distend the cecum, reflux back into the ileum is prevented by closure of the valve and reflex constriction of the sphincter.

GASTROILEAL REFLEX

At the end of the digestive period most of the residue of the meal has passed to the colon; only a small amount is left in the terminal ileum. Ingestion of the next meal empties the ileum via a sequence of events termed the gastroileal reflex. The reflex is initiated by the presence of food in the stomach, which enhances the contractile activity of the ileum and decreases the tone of the ileocecal sphincter. Although termed a reflex, there is virtually no evidence that these events are mediated by extrinsic nerves. The hormone gastrin, which is released from the antrum in response to food, may be responsible for this so-called reflex. Exogenous administration of gastrin, at physiologic doses, increases segmentation of the ileum and induces ileocecal sphincter relaxation.

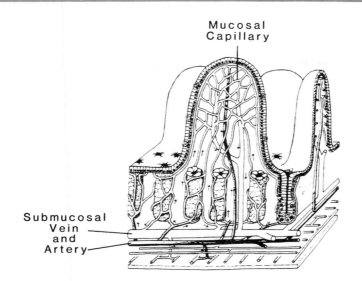

Mucosal
Capillary

Submucosal
Vein
and
Artery

FIGURE 7–31. Microvascular organization of the small intestine. (From Ohtani, O., Kikuta, A., Ohtsuka, A., Taguchi, T., and Murakami, T.: Microvasculature as studied by the microvascular corrosion casting/scanning electron microscope method. I. Endocrine and digestive system. Arch. Histol. Jpn., *46*:1–42, 1983.)

INTESTINO-INTESTINAL REFLEX

Another reflex called the intestino-intestinal reflex does require extrinsic innervation. This reflex is initiated by distention of a portion of the small intestine and results in the cessation of contractile activity in the remainder of the gut. The sympathetic nerves are the major component of this reflex arc, since bilateral section of the splanchnic nerves, but not vagotomy, abolishes it.

INTESTINAL CIRCULATION

Blood flow to the small intestine accounts for 10 to 15 per cent of resting cardiac output in the adult human. Blood is supplied to the small bowel almost entirely by the superior mesenteric artery; the celiac artery is a major contributor of blood to the duodenum, while the inferior mesenteric artery provides a small amount of blood to the terminal ileum. Experimental evidence indicates that there may be a gradient of blood flow (expressed per unit mass of tissue) from duodenum to ileum, with blood flow in the proximal bowel exceeding that of distal segments.

The mucosa, submucosa, and external muscle layers of the small intestine have discrete microvascular networks which are arranged as series and parallel coupled circuits (Fig. 7–31). The major arterial vessels supplying all three layers emanate from an arterial plexus located in the submucosa, just subjacent to the muscularis mucosae. Arterial vessels from the submucosal arterial plexus branch into capillaries in the longitudinal and circular muscle layers; the capillaries run parallel to the surrounding smooth muscle fibers. The microcirculation of the submucosa is sparse, except in the region of the duodenum that contains Brunner's glands. The arterial supply to the villus consists of one vessel, originating from the submucosal vascular plexus, which runs centrally in the lamina propria to the villus tip. At the villus tip, the arteriole branches into a fountain-like pattern of subepithelial capillaries. The capillaries, which are oriented parallel to the villus axis, empty into venules at different levels in the villus. The crypts of Lieberkühn are surrounded by a rich network of capillaries, which is fed by direct arterial connections from the submucosal vascular plexus. The venules draining the microvascular network of each layer empty into large veins located in submucosa.

The distribution of blood flow to the different layers of the small intestine has been estimated for a variety of conditions. Under resting conditions, approximately 75 per cent of total intestinal blood flow is distributed to the mucosa, 5 per cent to the submucosa, and 20 per cent to longitudinal and circular muscle layers. The villi receive approximately 60 per cent of the blood flow to the mucosal layer, with the crypts receiving the remainder. The relative distribution of blood flow to the different regions of the intestinal wall presumably reflects the varying metabolic demands of cells within each region. The highly metabolically active villus and crypt epithelium receive the largest proportion of flow, while the muscle layer, with its lower demand for oxygen, receives a somewhat lower fraction of total blood flow. The dependence of blood flow distribution on tissue demand is demonstrated by observations that blood flow is preferentially distributed to the mucosa during periods of enhanced nutrient absorption or electrolyte secretion, while increased intestinal motility is associated with blood flow redistribution to the muscle layers.

Blood flow to the small intestine increases by 30 to 130 per cent after a meal. The hyperemia is confined to that segment of bowel exposed to chyme, and the magnitude of the hyperemia is related to the type of food that is ingested. It appears that the hydrolytic products of food digestion are primarily responsible for the hyperemia in the duodenum and jejunum. Long-chain fatty acids (solubilized in bile) and glucose are the major luminal stimuli for the hyperemia. Although bile does not produce a hyperemia in the proximal intestine, it greatly increases blood flow in the terminal ileum. Bile salts, which are actively absorbed in the terminal ileum, are largely responsible for the bile-induced ileal hyperemia.

Several mechanisms have been proposed to explain the postprandial intestinal hyperemia. There is evidence that the mesenteric vasodilation during digestion involves a local cholinergic reflex. Cholecystokinin, which is released from mucosal endocrine cells when long-chain fatty acids or glucose is in the lumen, is a potent vasodilator at blood concentrations measured in portal venous blood after a meal. Since intestinal oxygen consumption rises in the postprandial period, metabolically linked vasodilators such as adenosine have been implicated in the hyperemia. Some constituents of chyme, once absorbed, can directly affect the intestinal vasculature. Bile salts directly produce vasodilation when infused into the arterial supply of the terminal ileum to achieve post-prandial blood concentrations. Interstitial osmolality also appears to play a major role in the functional intestinal hyperemia. The osmolality of the mucosal interstitium, in the vicinity of major resistance vessels, increases following food ingestion, owing to active transport of electrolytes and nutrients. The increased tissue osmolality and intestinal vasodilation are both temporally and quantitatively correlated. From the available evidence it appears unlikely that the postprandial intestinal hyperemia can be attributed to a single factor or mechanism.

A major function of intestinal capillaries and lymphatics is removal of absorbed nutrients and water from the mucosal interstitium. Both the capillaries and lacteals of the intestine are highly permeable to small solutes the size of glucose and amino acids; however, the capillaries remove virtually all of the absorbed water-soluble nutrients from the mucosal interstitium. The dominant role of the capillaries is due to the fact that blood flow is approximately 1000 times greater than lymph flow in the small intestine. The lymphatics play a more important role in removing large molecules (proteins) and particles (chylomicrons) from the mucosal interstitium. The lacteals are highly permeable to even the largest chylomicron (6000 Å diameter), while the fenestrated capillaries of the intestinal mucosa are relatively impermeable to proteins as small as albumin (75 Å diameter). Thus, the immunoglobulins (IgA), enzymes, and chylomicrons which are liberated into the mucosal interstitium gain access to the blood stream exclusively by way of lymph.

The process by which absorbed fluid is driven into the mucosal capillaries and lymphatics can be described in terms of the Starling capillary exchange equation:

$$\text{Net capillary fluid flux} = \text{Capillary hydraulic conductivity} \left[\text{Capillary-to-interstitium hydrostatic pressure gradient} - \left(\text{Capillary reflection coefficient} \times \text{Capillary-to-interstitium oncotic pressure gradient} \right) \right]$$

In the nonabsorbing small intestine (Fig. 7–32, upper), there is a small imbalance in the hydrostatic and oncotic forces acting across the capillary wall that favors net movement of fluid from blood to interstitium. Although small (0.3 mm Hg), this imbalance of forces is sufficient to cause significant leakage of fluid into the interstitium owing to the relatively high hydraulic conductivity of capillaries in the intestine. The rate of capillary filtration is balanced by an equal outflow of fluid via the lacteal.

When net water absorption is stimulated (Fig. 7–32, lower), mucosal interstitial volume rises, owing to accumulation of absorbed fluid in the subepithelial spaces. The interstitial volume expansion produces an increase in interstitial hydrostatic pressure (2.0 mm Hg) and a reduction in interstitial oncotic

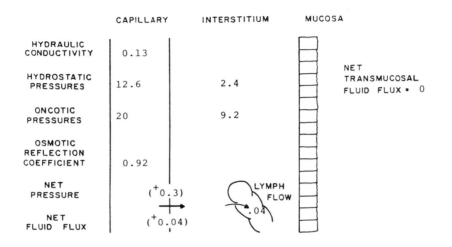

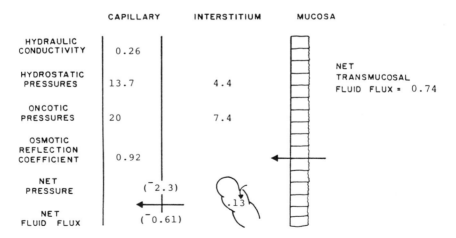

FIGURE 7–32. Summary of capillary and interstitial forces, capillary, lymphatic and mucosal water fluxes, and membrane coefficients in the nonabsorbing and absorbing intestine. (From Granger, D.N., Perry, M.A., Kvietys, P.R., and Taylor, A.E.: Capillary and interstitial forces during intestinal absorption. Gastroenterology, *86*:267, 1984.)

pressure (1.8 mm Hg). Associated with the changes in interstitial forces are an increase in capillary pressure (1.1 mm Hg, owing to the mesenteric vasodilation associated with absorption) and a doubling of capillary hydraulic conductivity due to perfusion of a larger number of capillaries. The absorption-induced changes in capillary and interstitial forces modify the balance of pressures across the capillaries to produce a net absorptive force of 2.3 mm Hg. This force, coupled to the elevated capillary hydraulic conductivity, drives approximately 80 per cent of the absorbed fluid into the mucosal capillaries. Intestinal lymph flow also increases during absorption because of the increased lymphatic filling resulting from the rise in interstitial hydrostatic pressure. The enhanced lymph flow removes the remaining 20 per cent of absorbed fluid from the mucosal interstitium. Thus, as a consequence of the reactions initiated by absorbed fluid entering the interstitium, two important changes occur: (1) filtering capillaries are converted to absorbing capillaries, and (2) the rate of lymph formation is increased. Consequently, absorbed fluid is removed from the mucosal interstitium via two routes, the capillaries and lacteals.

SMALL INTESTINAL PAIN

As with other hollow viscera, pain from the small intestine arises from stretching or distention. The nerves transmitting this pain are located in the muscle layer. Pain arising from the small intestine is felt in the central abdomen around the umbilicus. Pain from the distal ileum can be experienced in the right iliac fossa.

CLINICAL CORRELATIONS

Deranged small intestinal function is demonstrated by the condition of celiac disease (gluten-sensitive enteropathy), a disorder which affects the small intestinal mucosa in a diffuse continuous fashion. The disease is due to the toxic effect of gluten, a protein constituent of wheat flour, which results in a marked alteration in the architecture of the small intestinal mucosa in susceptible individuals. The histologic lesion in the full-blown condition is termed "total villous atrophy" and is most severe in the proximal small intestine, but may extend to involve the terminal ileum. The villi are absent; thus the mucosal surface is quite flat with the crypts opening onto the surface. The epithelium of the crypts is dividing very actively, but the enterocytes do not survive long enough to form villi. Since the acquisition of many important digestive enzymes such as disaccharidases and peptidases by the enterocyte occurs during its progress from crypt to villus tip, the surface epithelium in this disease is functionally immature. The clinical picture, a generalized malabsorption, is explicable both by the loss of absorptive surface area and a deficiency of mucosal enzymes involved in nutrient digestion and transport.

Patients often present with diarrhea and moderately increased stool fat. Abdominal cramps may occur; bacterial production of gas from unabsorbed nutrients may contribute to this. Various mechanisms are responsible for the diarrhea: malabsorption of nutrients causes osmotic effects with increased stool water; unabsorbed fatty acids are converted by enteric bacteria to hydroxy-fatty acids, which are powerful secretagogues in the colonic mucosa; and there is evidence that the abnormal small intestinal mucosa actively secretes water and electrolytes in this condition. If there is extensive involvement of the terminal ileum, malabsorption of bile acids occurs and a greater amount than the normal daily load of bile acids (approximately 300 mg) enters the colon. The bile acids and their bacterial derivatives such as deoxycholic acid have a secretagogue action on the colonic mucosa similar to hydroxy-fatty acids.

Although the primary physiologic defect in celiac disease is malabsorption, there is some evidence that cholecystokinin release from the diseased upper small intestinal mucosa may be defective; thus the pancreatic enzyme response to a meal is diminished and a component of maldigestion may result. The degree of steatorrhea in celiac disease is, however, seldom as great as that in severe pancreatic insufficiency, where lipolysis may be greatly impaired.

Since most foodstuffs are absorbed in the upper small intestine, a wide spectrum of nutritional deficiencies may be seen in celiac disease. Weight loss is common, and in severe cases hypoproteinemic edema may occur. Anemia due to malabsorption of iron or folic acid or both is very common and indeed may be the presenting and only feature of the disease. Vitamin B_{12} deficiency is seen only when the disease has extended to the terminal ileum. A variety of vitamin deficiencies may occur: night blindness (vitamin A), osteomalacia with pathologic fractures (vitamin D), and a bleeding tendency due to hypo-prothrombinemia (vitamin K). Oral lesions may be seen, some of which are the result of various B vitamin deficiencies. Bone disease may not be due simply to vitamin D deficiency. Calcium may be malabsorbed by the diseased mucosal cells, and unabsorbed fatty acids may sequester calcium in the form of insoluble soaps. It should be stressed that since there is a spectrum of severity of mucosal damage, this entire galaxy of deficiencies is seldom encountered in most cases where only one or two deficiencies may occur. Most patients have a gratifying response to the elimination of gluten (wheat flour and its various products) from the diet.

REFERENCES

Alpers, D.H.: Absorption of water-soluble vitamins, folate, minerals, and vitamin D. *In* Sleisenger, M.H., and Fordtran, J.S. (eds.): Gastrointestinal Disease: Pathophysiology, Diagnosis, Management, 3rd ed. Philadelphia, W.B. Saunders Co., 1983, pp. 830–842.

Barrowman, J.A.: Physiology of the Gastrointestinal Lymphatic System. London, Cambridge University Press, 1978.

Binder, H.J.: Absorption and secretion of water and electrolytes by small and large intestine. *In* Sleisenger, M.H., and Fordtran, J.S. (eds.): Gastrointestinal Disease: Pathophysiology, Diagnosis, Management, 3rd ed. Philadelphia, W.B. Saunders Co., 1983, pp. 811–829.

Binder, H.J.: Net fluid and electrolyte secretion: The pathologic basis for diarrhea. *In* Binder, H.J. (ed.): Mechanisms of Intestinal Secretion. New York, A.R. Liss, Inc., 1979, pp. 1–15.

Connell, A.M.: Dietary fiber. *In* Johnson, L.R. (ed.): Physiology of the Gastrointestinal Tract. New York, Raven Press, 1981, pp. 1291–1299.

Davenport, H.W.: Physiology of the Digestive Tract. Chicago, Year Book Medical Publishers, 1977.

Donaldson, R.M.: Intrinsic factor and the transport of cobalamin. In Johnson, L.R. (ed.): Physiology of the Gastrointestinal Tract. New York, Raven Press, 1981, pp. 641–658.

Field, M.: Secretion of electrolytes and water by mammalian small intestine. In Johnson, L.R. (ed.): Physiology of the Gastrointestinal Tract. New York, Raven Press, 1981, pp. 963–980.

Granger, D.N., and Barrowman, J.A.: Microcirculation of the alimentary tract. I. Physiology of transcapillary fluid and solute exchange. Gastroenterology, 84:846–868, 1983.

Granger, D.N., Kvietys, P.R., Parks, D.A., et al.: Intestinal blood flow: Relations to function. Sur. Dig. Dis., 1:217–228, 1983.

Gray, G.M.: Carbohydrate absorption and malabsorption. In Johnson, L.R. (ed.): Physiology of the Gastrointestinal Tract. New York, Raven Press, 1981, pp. 1063–1072.

Gray, G.M.: Mechanisms of digestion and absorption of food. In Sleisenger, M.H., and Fordtran, J.S. (eds.): Gastrointestinal Disease: Pathophysiology, Diagnosis, Management, 3rd ed. Philadelphia, W.B. Saunders Co., 1983, pp. 844–858.

Hendrix, T.T.: The absorptive function of the alimentary canal. In Mountcastle, V.B. (ed.): Medical Physiology. St. Louis, C.V. Mosby Co., 1980, pp. 1255–1288.

Jensen, D.: The Principles of Physiology. New York, Appleton-Century-Crofts, 1980.

Johnson, L.R. (ed.): Gastrointestinal Physiology. St. Louis, C.V. Mosby Co., 1981.

Johnson, L.R.: Regulation of gastrointestinal growth. In Johnson, L.R. (ed.): Physiology of the Gastrointestinal Tract. New York, Raven Press, 1981, pp. 169–196.

Kagnoff, M.F.: Immunology of the digestive system. In Johnson, L.R. (ed.): Physiology of the Gastrointestinal Tract. New York, Raven Press, 1981, pp, 1337–1359.

Patton, J.S.: Gastrointestinal lipid digestion. In Johnson, L.R. (ed.): Physiology of the Gastrointestinal Tract. New York, Raven Press, 1981, pp. 1123–1139.

Roman, C., and Gonella, J.: Extrinsic control of digestive tract motility. In Johnson, L.R. (ed.): Physiology of the Gastrointestinal Tract. New York, Raven Press, 1981, pp. 289–333.

Rose, R.C.: Intestinal absorption of water-soluble vitamins. In Johnson, L.R. (ed.): Physiology of the Gastrointestinal Tract. New York, Raven Press, 1981, pp. 1231–1241.

Rosenberg, I.H.: Intestinal absorption of folate. In Johnson, L.R. (ed.): Physiology of the Gastrointestinal Tract. New York, Raven Press, 1981, pp. 1221–1229.

Schultz, S.G.: Salt and water absorption by mammalian small intestine. In Johnson, L.R. (ed.): Physiology of the Gastrointestinal Tract. New York, Raven Press, 1981, pp. 983–989.

Sernka, T.J., and Jacobson, E.D.: Gastrointestinal Physiology. The Essentials. Baltimore, Williams and Wilkins, 1983.

Shepherd, A.P., and Granger, D.N.: Physiology of the Intestinal Circulation. New York, Raven Press, 1984.

Thomson, A.B.R., and Dietschy, J.M.: Intestinal lipid absorption: Major extracellular and intracellular events. In Johnson, L.R. (ed.): Physiology of the Gastrointestinal Tract. New York, Raven Press, 1981, pp. 1147–1194.

Trier, J.S., Krone, C.L., and Sleisenger, M.H.: Anatomy, embryology and developmental abnormalities of the small intestine and colon. In Sleisenger, M.H., and Fordtran, J.S. (eds.): Gastrointestinal Disease: Pathophysiology, Diagnosis, Management, 3rd ed. Philadelphia, W.B. Saunders Co., 1983, pp. 780–811.

Trier, J.S., and Modara, J.L.: Functional morphology of the mucosa of the small intestine. In Johnson, L.R. (ed.): Physiology of the Gastrointestinal Tract. New York, Raven Press, 1981, pp. 925–961.

Watson, D.W., and Sodeman, W.A.: The small intestine. In Sodeman, W.A., and Sodeman, T.M. (eds.): Pathologic Physiology: Mechanisms of Disease, 5th ed. Philadelphia, W.B. Saunders Co., 1974, pp. 734–766.

Weisbrodt, N.W.: Motility of the small intestine. In Johnson, L.R. (ed.): Physiology of the Gastrointestinal Tract. New York, Raven Press, 1981, pp. 411–443.

Weisbrodt, N.W.: Patterns of intestinal motility. Annu. Rev. Physiol., 43:21–31, 1981.

Wood, J.D.: Intrinsic neural control of intestinal motility. Annu. Rev. Physiol., 43:33–51, 1981.

Wood, J.D.: Physiology of the enteric nervous system. In Johnson, L.R. (ed.): Physiology of the Gastrointestinal Tract. New York, Raven Press, 1981, pp. 1–37.

Although the large intestine is generally perceived as a simple storage depot for fecal material, it is now recognized as a digestive and absorptive organ of significant import. One of the most important functions of the large intestine is to absorb most of the 1.5 liters of water and electrolytes which escape absorption in the small bowel each day. In addition, the large number of bacteria in the colon transform food residues and dietary fiber into substances of caloric value, which are subsequently absorbed. The mixing and propulsive activities of the colonic smooth muscle are designed to facilitate absorption by continuously re-exposing "chyme" to the absorptive cells. When "chyme" has been sufficiently dehydrated and the residual material reaches the rectum, the urge to defecate is felt. The process of defecation is complex and involves both voluntary and involuntary reflexes. The voluntary component of the defecation reflex allows for discretionary fecal elimination.

8

THE LARGE INTESTINE

ANATOMY

The large intestine extends from the ileocecal junction to the anus. It can be anatomically subdivided into the cecum (and its appendix), ascending colon, transverse colon, descending colon, sigmoid colon, rectum, and anus (Fig. 8–1). The large bowel is approximately 125 cm long in vivo, which is much shorter than the small intestine. The "large" intestine derives its name from the characteristically widened external diameter, relative to the small bowel. Although the proximal large intestine is twice as wide as the small bowel, the more distal portions of the colon have a caliber similar to that of the small bowel. The cecum is the widest portion of the colon, being about 8.5 cm in diameter, while the diameter is narrowed to 2.0 to 2.5 cm at the level of the sigmoid colon. The most striking feature of the large intestine is the presence of haustra (recesses), which give it a sacculated appearance. Haustra are more prevalent in the proximal portions of the large intestine.

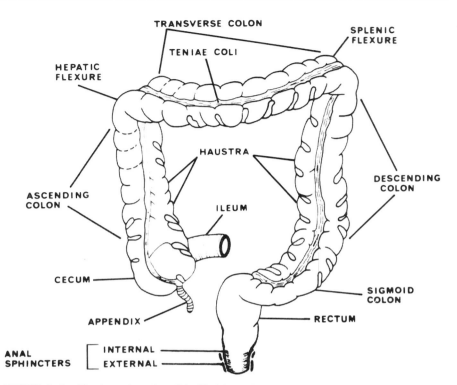

FIGURE 8–1. The large intestine. (Modified from Jensen, D.: The Principles of Physiology. New York, Appleton-Century-Crofts, 1976, p. 843.)

The wall of the colon, like that of the small intestine, is divided into four layers: serosa, muscularis externa, submucosa, and mucosa. However, there are several anatomic specializations in the colon which distinguish this portion of the gut from the small intestine.

Serosa

The squamous epithelium of the colonic serosa is studded by elongated protrusions of the peritoneum containing fat. These structures, called *appendices epiploicae*, are larger and more prevalent in the distal portion of the colon. The serosal layer is absent at the level of the rectum.

Muscularis Externa

As in the small bowel, the muscle coat of the colon consists of an outer longitudinal layer and an inner circular layer. However, the longitudinal muscle layer of the colon is not distributed evenly around its circumference but is concentrated into three bands called the *teniae coli*. The bands, which are 0.8 cm wide, are separated by a thin sheet of longitudinal muscle. The three teniae coli, which are situated equidistantly around the circumference of the colon, contribute to the sacculated appearance of this organ. Haustral formation is also facilitated by the elongation of the circular muscle so that the inner muscle layer appears to bulge outward between the teniae coli. The bulge is interrupted at various sites by constricted bands of circular muscle, the plicae circulares. The size and shape of the haustrations are not fixed but depend on the contractile activity of the circular and longitudinal muscle layers. At the distal portion of the sigmoid colon, the teniae coli broaden and converge so that the longitudinal muscle is one uniform and continuous sheet covering the rectum.

Nerve plexuses lie in the connective tissue bordering the muscle layers. The myenteric plexus is located between the circular and longitudinal muscles. The neurons of the myenteric plexus are concentrated beneath the teniae coli and are more sparsely distributed between them. The submucous plexus lies beneath the circular muscle layer and is more prominent in the rectum than elsewhere along the colon.

Mucosa

The mucosa of the colon is characterized by a relatively smooth surface. The anatomic modifications of the colonic mucosa which increase its surface area are not as distinctive as those of the small intestine. The colonic mucosal surface is thrown into irregular folds (plicae semilunares), which are less prominent than the plicae circulares of the small bowel mucosa. The mucosa of the colon is devoid of villi, and the microvilli of the colonic absorptive cells are less abundant than their counterparts in the small intestine. Nonetheless, the plicae semilunares and microvilli increase the surface area of the colonic mucosa by as much as 10 to 15 times that predicted for a simple cylinder.

The colonic mucosa is partitioned into three layers: the muscularis mucosae, the lamina propria, and the epithelium. The muscularis mucosa is a layer of smooth muscle approximately 8 to 12 cells thick, which separates the submucosa from the lamina propria of the mucosa. The lamina propria provides structural support for the epithelium; within its connective tissue lie the blood vessels and lymphatics.

The lamina propria of the large intestine contains numerous T lymphocytes, macrophages, plasma cells, and occasional lymphoid nodules which protrude into the submucosa. The plasma cells secrete immunoglobulins (primarily IgA), and the lymphoid tissue can mount an immune response. The immune function of the colon is particularly important because of its extensive bacterial flora. The lamina propria of the fetal colon is devoid of immune cells. Only after birth, when the colon is colonized by bacteria, do the lymphoid and plasma cells appear.

EPITHELIAL CELLS

Although the mucosal surface of the colon is devoid of villi, there are numerous crypts (about 0.7 mm deep) extending from the flat absorptive surface to the muscularis mucosa. The cells in the crypts and on the mucosal surface are somewhat similar to those found in the small intestine. The goblet and endocrine cells of the colonic mucosa are morphologically indistinguishable from their counterparts in the small bowel (see Fig. 7–4). The goblet cells, with their mucus-laden granules, are more prominent in the colon than in the small intestine. The large number of goblet cells in the colon minimizes the frictional interaction between the semisolid feces and the mucosal surface. There are fewer endocrine cells in the colon, and they differ from those in the small intestine only in regard to the type of hormones secreted (see Fig. 1–2).

The epithelia in the lower half of the colonic crypts consist primarily of undifferentiated cells which ultimately give rise to the goblet, endocrine, and absorptive cells. The undifferentiated cells migrate up the crypt as they proliferate and mature. Upon reaching the mucosal surface, they degenerate and eventually slough off into the lumen. The kinetics of epithelial cell proliferation, migration, and extrusion are slightly slower in the colon than in the small intestine, requiring approximately four to seven days for a complete turnover.

Mucosal Growth and Adaptation

The proliferative activity of the colonic mucosa is largely dependent on lumen contents. Food deprivation results in a reduction of mucosal surface area in the colon, primarily as a result of decreased cell proliferation in the crypts. Reinstitution of feeding with a bulk-free diet does not alleviate the mucosal atrophy, since the nutrients are almost completely absorbed by the small intestine. If, however, bulk is added to the diet, the mucosal surface area, as well as cell proliferation kinetics, is returned to normal. Extensive surgical resection of the small bowel, which is associated with enhanced delivery of unabsorbed nutrients to the colon, increases colonic weight, length, and circumference. Feeding nonmetabolizable bulk to experimental animals results in hypertrophy of the proximal colon and an increase in its solute transport capacity. Thus, in contrast to the small intestine, luminal nutrients are of secondary importance in maintaining cell turnover rate and growth in the colon. The presence of bacteria in the lumen is also important in maintaining a normally functioning mucosa, for in their absence there is a decrease in cell proliferation. Antrectomy (eliminating endogenous gastrin) results in atrophy of the colonic mucosa, an effect which can be reversed by exogenously administered gastrin. Therefore, gastrin may also play a role in the regulation of colonic growth.

WATER AND ELECTROLYTE TRANSPORT

Water Transport

The large intestine normally absorbs a smaller quantity of fluid than does the small intestine, but it does so much more efficiently. Approximately 1.5 liters of fluid enter the large intestine of the adult human each day. Ninety per cent of this fluid load is absorbed, leaving only 100 to 150 ml of water to be excreted in stools (Fig. 8–2A). The maximum capacity of the human colon to absorb water may be as great as 4.5 liters per day. Provided that the rate of entry of fluid into the colon is less than the maximum absorptive capacity, net fluid secretion can occur in the small intestine, but diarrhea (increased fecal water excretion) will not occur (Fig. 8–2B). However, when ileocecal flow exceeds the absorptive capacity of the colon (Fig. 8–2C), or if there is actual colonic fluid secretion (Fig. 8–2D), diarrhea will ensue. Therefore, the capacity of the colon to absorb water is critical in determining whether or not there is diarrhea when either the small or large bowel is diseased.

Water absorption in the large bowel is coupled to, and dependent on, solute (electrolyte) absorption. The coupling of solute and water fluxes in the colon can be explained in terms of the standing osmotic gradient theory. An osmotic gradient is established between the lumen and lateral intercellular space by active transport of electrolytes into the latter compartment. The osmotic gradient draws water across the tight junctions and through the cell into the intercellular space (see Fig. 1–13). Unlike the small intestine and gallbladder, in which absorbed electrolytes are accompanied by an isosmotic equivalent of water, the large bowel generates a hypertonic absorbate. The human colon transports water against osmotic gradients of up to 50 mOsm per liter, indicating that a large osmotic gradient is needed to drive water through the colonic epithelial barrier. This observation is explained by the relatively high mucosal resistance (compared with jejunum and ileum) in the colon. The effective pore size of the colonic mucosa is approximately 2.3 Å (radius), which is significantly smaller than the 8 Å and 4 Å pore radii predicted for the jejunum and ileum, respectively. The relative tightness of colonic epithelia accounts for the ability of the colon to generate a hypertonic absorbate and to generate rather large concentration differences for electrolytes between lumen and plasma. This is explained by the fact that passive water movement into the intercellular spaces proceeds more slowly, owing to high resistance, than does electrolyte transport. Another functional consequence of the low permeability of the colonic epithelium is a larger spontaneous potential difference across the epithelial layer than those measured in jejunum and ileum.

Although we have employed the terms colon and large intestine interchangeably to describe that segment of bowel that begins at the cecum and ends at the anus, there are important differences in transport function among the different regions of the large intestine. Studies in humans and experimental animals indicate that the rate of water absorption is greater in the proximal

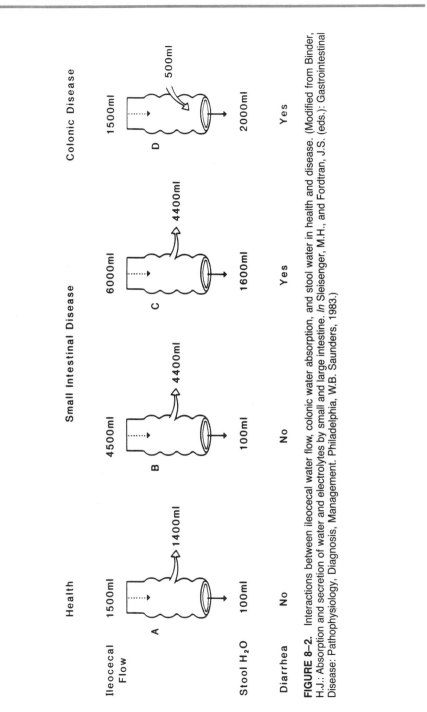

FIGURE 8–2. Interactions between ileocecal water flow, colonic water absorption, and stool water in health and disease. (Modified from Binder, H.J.: Absorption and secretion of water and electrolytes by small and large intestine. *In* Sleisenger, M.H., and Fordtran, J.S. (eds.): Gastrointestinal Disease: Pathophysiology, Diagnosis, Management. Philadelphia, W.B. Saunders, 1983.)

large bowel (cecum to transverse colon) than in the distal segment (transverse colon to rectum). The cecum is the most permeable region of the large bowel (comparable to the ileum), whereas the rectal mucosa is the least permeable. Thus, the ability of the colon to generate a hypertonic absorbate increases in the aboral direction so that the final fecal water is hypotonic with respect to plasma.

Electrolyte Transport

SODIUM

The large intestine is more efficient at conserving sodium than is the small intestine. Approximately 150 mEq of sodium enter the colon each day, yet only 1 to 5 mEq are lost in stools. The 95 per cent or greater efficiency of the colon in conserving sodium compares with the 75 per cent efficiency of the small bowel. Furthermore, the colon can absorb net sodium even when the luminal concentration is as low as 30 mEq per liter, whereas net sodium absorption in the jejunum does not occur when luminal sodium concentration falls below 130 mEq per liter. The differences in efficiency of sodium transport between the small and large bowels result from the relatively higher permeability of small bowel mucosa to sodium. The small intestine cannot absorb sodium against a concentration gradient because of a large permeability-associated plasma-to-lumen movement ("back leak") of sodium.

Sodium absorption in the human colon is an active, electrogenic process (Fig. 8–3). Sodium crosses the apical membrane of colonic epithelium by simple diffusion through water-filled pores or channels. Inasmuch as the mucosal cell interior is electronegative (-30 mv) with respect to the lumen (0 mv), and the intracellular sodium concentration is one tenth the lumen concentration, sodium moves into the cell down both electrical and concentration gradients. Sodium exit from the cell is directed against steep concentration (14 mM to 140 mM) and electrical (-30 mv to $+20$ mv) gradients. A sodium-potassium exchange pump, located at the basolateral membrane, is responsible for the "uphill" transport of sodium out of the cell. The energy required for the sodium pump is derived from ATP hydrolysis via the enzyme, Na^+, K^+-ATPase. Sodium exit from the cell is inhibited by low extracellular potassium concentrations or ouabain, an inhibitor of Na^+, K^+-ATPase.

Electrogenic transport is probably the only process responsible for sodium absorption in the human colon. In contrast to the small intestine, glucose and other nonelectrolytes do not stimulate colonic sodium absorption, indicating that a nonelectrolyte-stimulated absorptive process does not exist in the colon. Passive absorption of sodium secondary to bulk flow of water (convection) is negligible in the colon owing to the tightness of the mucosal epithelium. While neutral sodium chloride absorption has been demonstrated in the colon of some experimental animals, this mechanism is not present in humans.

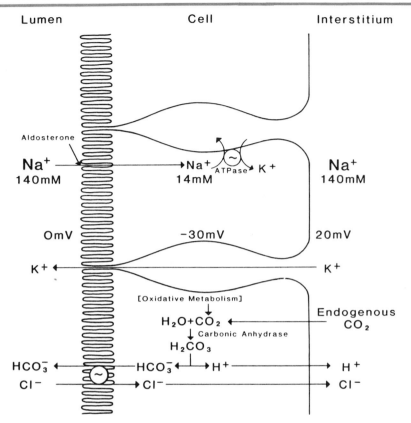

Lumen   Cell   Interstitium

FIGURE 8–3. Mechanisms involved in colonic transport of sodium, potassium, chloride, and bicarbonate ions.

POTASSIUM

Approximately 10 mEq of potassium enter the healthy human large intestine each day, while 5 to 15 mEq K^+ are lost in the stools over the same period of time. Whether the colon absorbs or secretes potassium is largely dependent upon its concentration in the lumen; net secretion occurs when the luminal concentration is less than 15 mEq per liter, but higher lumen concentrations are associated with net potassium absorption. These observations are consistent with passive movement along electrochemical gradients. Inasmuch as luminal potassium concentration is usually less than 15 mEq per liter, net secretion normally occurs (Fig. 8–3). The tight junctions between colonic epithelium are highly permeable to potassium ions. This high permeability, coupled to the transepithelial electrical potential difference (lumen negative with respect to plasma), allows potassium to diffuse readily from plasma to lumen.

While passive diffusion across tight junctions is the primary mechanism of potassium transport in the colon, a small portion of the secretory potassium flux is due to active transcellular transport. For this process, potassium is transported into the cell at the basolateral membrane by the Na^+-K^+ pump, creating a high intracellular potassium concentration (80 mM). As a result of the high intracellular concentration, potassium diffuses out of the cell at the apical membrane and into the lumen. This process normally produces only a small secretory potassium flux, because the apical cell membrane is essentially impermeable to this ion. Nonetheless, agents or conditions which increase the permeability of the apical membrane to potassium may increase potassium secretory rate via this process.

Hormonal Control of Colonic Sodium and Potassium Transport

Mineralocorticoids and glucocorticoids are both known to stimulate sodium absorption and potassium secretion in the mammalian colon. Aldosterone, at concentrations secreted endogenously in response to sodium depletion or potassium loading, significantly alters sodium and potassium fluxes across the colonic mucosa, so that the stool sodium concentration decreases to one tenth while the potassium concentration doubles. Therapeutic doses of glucocorticoids are required to produce the same effects; such doses are often used clinically to treat many gastrointestinal diseases. The mechanisms of adrenocorticosteroid action on colonic transport appear to involve an increase in the permeability of the apical membrane to sodium and potassium as well as an enhancement of Na^+,K^+-ATPase activity. The increased apical membrane permeability and enhanced sodium-potassium pump activity both tend to enhance sodium absorption and potassium secretion. In contrast to the colon, the small intestine is insensitive to mineralocorticoids.

CHLORIDE AND BICARBONATE

The mammalian colon is highly efficient in absorbing chloride ions. Approximately 100 mEq of chloride enter the human colon each day, yet only 1 to 2 mEq are lost in stools. Net chloride absorption occurs even when the luminal chloride concentration is as low as 25 mEq per liter, indicating that it is actively absorbed. Based on observations that (1) chloride absorption is electrically silent (does not generate an electrical potential), (2) a reciprocal relation exists between the disappearance of chloride from the lumen and the appearance of bicarbonate, and (3) carbonic anhydrase inhibitors block chloride absorption and bicarbonate secretion, an anion exchange process has been invoked to explain chloride absorption in the human colon (Fig. 8–3). According to this concept, carbon dioxide (derived from blood and cellular metabolism) reacts with water in the presence of carbonic anhydrase (which is present in high concentrations in the colonic mucosa) to form carbonic acid. Hydrogen ions that are produced by the dissociation of carbonic acid exit the cell at the basolateral membrane, while bicarbonate ions are transported out of the cell (secreted) via a carrier protein at the apical membrane in exchange for chloride

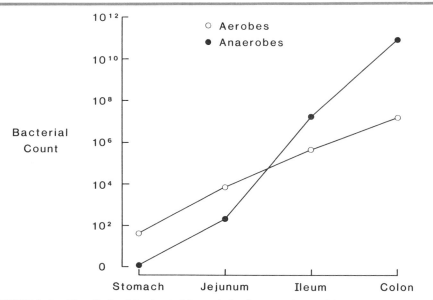

FIGURE 8–4. Magnitude of the bacterial population in stomach, small intestine, and colon.

ions. Chloride exit from the cell involves a passive process that does not require energy. Thus, the anion exchange process allows the colon to absorb chloride and to secrete bicarbonate. The concentration of HCO_3^- in fecal water exceeds that in plasma, accounting for the alkalinity of fecal water.

DIGESTION AND ABSORPTION OF FOOD RESIDUES

Although the human colon is incapable of absorbing the principal break-down products of foodstuff (glucose, peptides, amino acids, long-chain fatty acids) in the form that they are delivered by the ileum, there are a large number of microbes in the colon that transform these and other food residues to substances which can be absorbed. An understanding of the extensive colonic microflora is necessary to appreciate their influence on digestion and transport.

Bacteriology of the Colon

The microflora of the human colon consists of both aerobic and anaerobic bacteria, with individual colons harboring more than 400 different bacterial species. The total bacterial count in the colon greatly exceeds that of the stomach and small intestine (Fig. 8–4). Anaerobic bacteria predominate in the colon, exceeding aerobic species by a factor of 10^2 to 10^4. *Bacteroides* and *Eubacterium* are the most common anaerobes in the colon, while *E. coli*, enterococci, and *Lactobacillus* are the most prevalent aerobes. The extremely large number of bacteria in the colon is exemplified by the fact that nearly one third the dry weight of feces consists of bacteria. The rate of bacterial multiplication is on the order of one to four divisions per day. A major factor contributing to the luxuriant flora in the colon is the low peristaltic activity. Normal peristalsis in the small bowel is sufficient to prevent bacterial overgrowth; however, conditions which abolish peristalsis are associated with a dense, colon-like bacterial flora. The microflora of the colon is relatively stable in regard to both absolute and relative amounts of bacteria, and even changes in diet such as dietary fiber supplements have little effect on the flora.

Carbohydrate Digestion

Carbohydrates that are not absorbed in the small intestine (e.g., dietary fiber), as well as the carbohydrate component of mucus, are transformed into acetic, propionic, and butyric acids by bacteria within the lumen of the colon. The short-chain fatty acids produced by carbohydrate fermentation account for over 50 per cent of the total anion content of human feces. The luminal concentration of short-chain fatty acids increases markedly approximately two hours after a meal. Luminal bicarbonate neutralizes a significant fraction of the acid load generated by these volatile short-chain fatty acids, resulting in the production of carbon dioxide and water. The human large intestine absorbs significant quantities of short-chain fatty acids, primarily by nonionic diffusion. Once absorbed, the fatty acids either are metabolized to ketone bodies by colonic epithelium or are transported via the portal vein to other tissues (e.g., liver) where they can be utilized as an energy source. While the nutritional importance of short-chain fatty acid absorption remains uncertain for man, it is well recognized that some ruminants obtain 70 per cent of their energy requirements from short-chain fatty acid production and absorption in the forestomach. A potentially important physiologic effect of short-chain fatty acids in the human colon is augmentation of sodium, potassium, and water absorption. The enhanced sodium and potassium absorption is presumed to result from ionic diffusion of sodium and potassium salts of short-chain fatty acids.

Lipid Digestion

Humans can normally excrete up to 5 grams of fat per day, yet only 50 per cent of fecal fat is of dietary origin. Although the degree of lipid digestion that occurs in the human large bowel remains uncertain, it is recognized that colonic bacteria possess exocellular lipases which exhibit activities and specificities similar to the lipases found in pancreatic juice. Most of the microbial lipases selectively hydrolyze fatty acid esters only at the 1 and 3 positions of the triglyceride molecule (like pancreatic lipase). Colonic microbes also have enzymes which metabolize long-chain fatty acids. Up to 25 per cent of total fecal fatty acids are hydroxylated by bacteria in the colon. Hydroxylated fatty acids such as hydroxystearic acid (a product of microbial hydration of oleic acid) can exert a profound influence on colonic electrolyte and water transport. These substances inhibit net absorption of water and electrolytes by the colon and induce net secretion (and diarrhea) at high luminal concentrations.

Virtually all of the cholesterol entering the colon is excreted in feces. A small proportion of the cholesterol is metabolized by colonic bacteria to coprostanol and coprostanone, both of which are poorly soluble and unavailable for absorption.

Bile Acid Metabolism

Bile acids which are not absorbed in the ileum enter the colon, where they are extensively metabolized by the microflora. The number of bile acid metabolites produced by colonic bacteria is enormous. The degradative reactions include deconjugation, dehydroxylation, desulfation, oxidation, reduction, and even desaturation of the steroid ring. The products of these reactions are more lipid-soluble than the substrates, which facilitates passive bile acid absorption in the colon. It is estimated that 50 mg per day of bile acids are passively absorbed in the human colon, primarily as a result of microbial degradation.

The normal daily fecal loss of bile acids ranges between 300 and 500 mg. Fecal loss of bile acids is influenced by a number of factors related to diet. An increased fat or dietary fiber load to the colon is associated with an increased fecal loss of bile acids. Both fat and fiber sequester bile acids in the lumen of the colon and thereby interfere with their absorption. The ideal diet for bile acid conservation in the colon is one that has no solid residue to act as a sequestrant; such a diet is used prior to large bowel surgery, and it is associated with low fecal loss of bile acids.

Vitamin K

Colonic bacteria can synthesize the K vitamins; enough of this is normally absorbed to meet the daily requirements in humans. Excessive use of laxatives, together with a nonabsorbable antibiotic, can produce vitamin K deficiency.

Ammonia Metabolism in the Colon

Approximately 25 per cent of urea synthesized in the liver reaches the gastrointestinal tract by diffusion from the blood. Bacterial urease in the colon converts it to ammonia, which diffuses readily across the colonic mucosa into portal venous blood and returns to the liver, where it is resynthesized to urea. Since NH_4^+ does not diffuse across the mucosa, some trapping of NH_3 in the colon occurs if its contents are acidified. The absorption of NH_3 from the colon is believed to be of importance in the raised blood ammonia levels of patients with portal-systemic shunting in liver disease.

TABLE 8–1.   Composition of Gastrointestinal Gas

	Stomach (%)	Intestine (%)	Flatus (%)
Nitrogen	79	64	61.2
Carbon dioxide	4	14	8.1
Hydrogen	0	19	19.8
Methane	0	8.8	7.3
Oxygen	17	0.7	3.6

From Levitt, M.D., Bond, J.H., and Levitt, D.G.: Gastrointestinal gas. *In* Johnson, L.R. (ed.): Physiology of the Gastrointestinal Tract, Vol. 2. New York, Raven Press, 1981.

COLONIC GAS

The gastrointestinal tract of normal individuals contains approximately 100 ml of gas (Table 8–1). There are four major sources of gastrointestinal gas: (1) swallowed air, (2) carbon dioxide liberated from the reaction of hydrogen and bicarbonate ions in the gut lumen, (3) volatile metabolites produced by intestinal bacteria, and (4) diffusion of gas from blood to lumen. The latter two sources contribute significantly to gas production in the colon. A variety of bacteria in the colon produce hydrogen gas, methane, and carbon dioxide through metabolism of unabsorbed polysaccharides (dietary fiber) and other food residues. Ingestion of fermentable substrates results in negligible hydrogen gas production in the small intestine (Fig. 8–5). In contrast, delivery of fermentable substrates to the colon leads to the production of appreciable volumes of hydrogen gas. This difference in the ability of the small and large bowel to produce H_2 largely reflects the greater number and types of bacteria in the large intestine. Ingestion of certain foods, particularly beans, which are rich in undigestable oligosaccharides (e.g., stachyose, raffinose) leads to massive increases in the H_2 content of flatus (air expelled through the anus). The rate of excretion

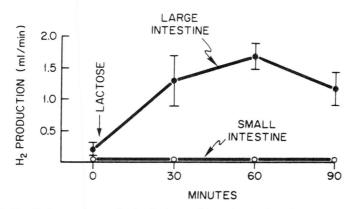

FIGURE 8–5.   Hydrogen gas production in the small bowel and colon of normal subjects before and after intraluminal infusion of 2 grams of lactose. (From Levitt, M.D., Bond, J.H., and Levitt, D.G.: Gastrointestinal gas. *In* Johnson, L.R. (ed.): Physiology of the Gastrointestinal Tract. New York, Raven Press, 1981.)

of hydrogen gas in the breath can be used as a sensitive test for carbohydrate malabsorption, inasmuch as some of the H_2 produced in the colon is absorbed into the blood and eventually eliminated by the lungs.

Methane and carbon dioxide are also produced by colonic bacteria and eliminated in flatus. Methane gas that is produced in the colon becomes entrapped in feces, causing the stool to float in the toilet bowel (the floating or sinking tendency of a stool is determined almost entirely by its gas content). It is interesting to note that the ability of an individual to produce appreciable quantities of methane is familial. When both parents are CH_4 producers, there is a 95 per cent incidence of production in the siblings, whereas the incidence is only 5 per cent when neither parent is a CH_4 producer. Since children raised in close quarters (but with no common genetics) also have the same CH_4-producing status, the familial tendency may be early environmental rather than hereditary.

Nitrogen is the predominant component of colonic gas in normal individuals. The nitrogen gas found in the lumen of the colon (and flatus) is derived from diffusion of the gas down a partial pressure gradient from blood to lumen. A reduced partial pressure for nitrogen in the lumen results from bacterial production of CO_2, H_2, and CH_4 in the lumen.

It is estimated that 1 to 1.5 liters of flatus are passed in a 24-hour period, at a rate of about 14 times a day. The passage of flatus normally accompanies the increased motor activity associated with food ingestion. Flatulence begins about one hour after the start of a meal and lasts for 20 minutes or more.

MOTILITY

Intrinsic Influences

The contractile activity of the colon is dictated by the basal electrical rhythm or slow waves of its external muscle layers. The frequency of the slow waves determines the maximal number of contractions possible, while the number of spike potentials generated during the depolarization phase determines the strength of the contractions. The slow-wave frequency of colonic smooth muscle is highly variable and is not characterized by a proximal-to-distal frequency gradient. The dominant slow-wave frequency is 11 cycles per minute, and it occurs along a frequency plateau that extends from the proximal portion of the transverse colon to the descending colon. The slow-wave frequency in the ascending colon, cecum, and sigmoid colon is generally lower than that observed on the frequency plateau. The highest recorded slow-wave frequency in the entire gastrointestinal tract occurs at the level of the rectum (17 cycles per min). This pattern of slow-wave frequency is the basis for the erratic and slow transit of "chyme" through the colon.

Neural and Humoral Influences

The neurons of the myenteric plexus exert a net inhibitory influence on colonic smooth muscle cells. Their tonic inhibitory nature is exemplified by a

TABLE 8–2.   Colonic Motility

Type of Movement	Frequency of Occurrence		Distance Traveled	Rate (cm/min)
	At Rest (%)	Postprandial (%)		
Haustral shuttling	38	13	0	0
Haustral propulsion	36	57	5–10 cm	2.5
Haustral retropulsion	30	52	5–20 cm	2.5
Multihaustral propulsion	9	17	Variable	2.5–5
Peristalsis	6	8	18–20 cm	1–2
Mass	Rare	12	≥ 30 cm	5–35

condition in which the myenteric plexus is absent (Hirschsprung's disease). In Hirschsprung's disease, the aganglionic colonic segment is tonically constricted. The myenteric plexus of the colon also contains excitatory cholinergic neurons as well as various peptidergic neurons containing VIP, substance P, enkephalins, and somatostatin.

Axons from both branches of the autonomic nervous system impinge on the neurons of the myenteric plexus. The parasympathetic supply to the proximal colon is by way of the vagus, whereas that to the distal colon is by way of the pelvic nerves. Although the parasympathetic nerves have an excitatory influence on colonic smooth muscle, different types of contractions are elicited during nerve stimulation. Vagal stimulation induces segmental contractions in the proximal colon; pelvic nerve stimulation produces tonic propulsive contractions in the distal colon. The sympathetic supply to the proximal colon is derived from the splanchnic nerves emerging from the superior mesenteric ganglia. The lumbar nerves, which originate from the inferior mesenteric ganglia, supply sympathetic nerves to the distal colon. Stimulation of either the splanchnic or lumbar nerves causes the colonic musculature to relax.

The extrinsic nerves are involved in several reflexes which alter colonic motility. The sympathetic branches mediate the reflex inhibition of colonic motility initiated by distention of the small intestine (intestino-colic reflex) or colon (colo-colic reflex). The parasympathetic (pelvic) nerves are involved in reflexes associated with defecation.

Various substances of gastrointestinal origin alter colonic motility. In general, their effects on colonic smooth muscle are similar to those observed in the small intestine (see Table 7–7).

Patterns of Contractions

The various types of contractions which occur in the large bowel during the interdigestive and digestive period are listed in Table 8–2. The most commonly observed motor patterns are haustral shuttling and propulsive contractions (Fig. 8–6). Contractions of the circular muscle in the proximal and mid-

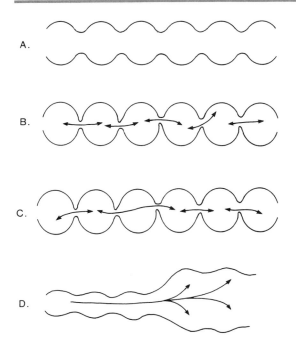

FIGURE 8-6. The process of haustral shuttling and propulsion. *A,* A quiescent segment of colon. *B,* Haustral shuttling with no net movement of chyme. *C,* Haustral shuttling with propulsion of chyme from one haustrum to another. *D,* Multihaustral propulsion with movement of chyme through several haustra.

colon are primarily responsible for the formation of haustra. At any given locus, haustrations are formed and disappear in a random fashion owing to segmental contractions of the circular muscle. These contractions lead to haustral shuttling if the lumen contents are simply displaced in both directions, and there is little or no movement. Extensions of this simple shuttling activity are haustral propulsion and retropulsion. Haustral propulsion occurs when adjacent haustra contract sequentially, so that the contents of a single haustrum are displaced into the adjacent segment and subsequently to another haustrum downstream. Haustral retropulsion occurs when the sequential haustral contractions move "chyme" orally from one haustrum to another. Multihaustral propulsion is accomplished by the simultaneous contraction of several haustra which empty their contents into several adjacent haustra downstream. Multihaustral retropulsion does not usually occur. In general, all of the aforementioned segmental contractions, involving either a single haustrum or several haustra, occur with increasing frequency after a meal (Table 8-2).

Peristaltic contractions occur much less frequently than the segmental type of motor activity. Peristalsis in the colon is a similar phenomenon to that observed in the small intestine, i.e., a propagated wave of contraction preceded by an area of relaxation which moves "chyme." However, peristaltic waves can move colonic contents 18 to 20 cm, a distance ten times greater than that traveled by peristaltic waves in the small intestine. Peristaltic contractions in the colon can move either aborally or orally. A peristaltic wave which moves

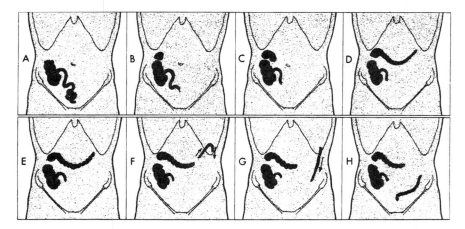

FIGURE 8–7.   The movements of the large intestine after a meal, illustrating the mass propulsion of chyme. The subject had a breakfast containing barium sulfate at 7 A.M. At 12 noon the barium shadow was visible in the terminal ileum, cecum, and ascending colon (*A*). He then ate a meal, which resulted in the movement of chyme from the ileum into the colon (*B*). Subsequently a portion of chyme was moved into the transverse colon, and haustral (segmental) contractions mixed the chyme (*C* to *E*). About 5 minutes later the shadow became elongated, and a portion passed around the splenic flexure (*F*) and down the descending colon (*G*) to the level of the sigmoid colon (*H*). (Adapted from Davenport, H.W.: Physiology of the Digestive Tract, 4th ed. Chicago, Year Book Medical Publishers, 1977, p. 78.)

colonic contents over long distances (30 cm or more) is referred to as "mass propulsion." These peristaltic waves usually begin in the transverse colon and can move chyme as far down as the rectum (Fig. 8–7). Mass propulsion or peristalsis is rarely observed in the fasting individual but usually occurs soon after ingestion of a meal.

Effects of Feeding on Colonic Motility

The contractile activity of the colon increases after feeding (Table 8–2). The amount of food ingested does not appear to influence the response. However, the intensity of the postprandial contractile activity is directly related to the caloric content of the ingested food. Of the three major classes of nutrients, fats appear to be the most important determinant of the postprandial response. High protein or carbohydrate meals do not substantially alter colonic motility. The postprandial motor response involves a cholinergic component, since oral administration of anticholinergic agents prevents the response to a meal. Cholinergic involvement in this reflex may be related to the ability of acetylcholine to release gastrointestinal hormones. Both gastrin and cholecystokinin are released after meals, and both have been implicated in the postprandial motor response based on their ability to contract colonic smooth muscle. The term *gastrocolic reflex* has been applied to the enhancement of colonic motor activity produced by ingestion of food.

The type of contractile activity induced by feeding is different in various segments of the colon. In the cecum and ascending colon, the major sites of fluid and electrolyte absorption, the movements are segmental in nature, with haustral shuttling being the predominant activity. Propulsive and retropulsive haustral contractions, as well as peristaltic contractions, are commonly observed at the level of the transverse colon following a meal. Since the slow wave frequency is higher in this region than in either the proximal or distal segments, "chyme" moves both aborally and orally. Luminal material that is propelled from the transverse colon to the cecum mixes with the fresh chyme that passes into the cecum as a result of the gastroileal reflex. Cecal contents are prevented from refluxing into the ileum by the ileocecal valve and sphincter (see Fig. 7–30). The net effect of postprandial motor activity in the proximal portion of the colon is to retain and mix "chyme" and prolong the time available for absorption. The propulsive activity of the more distal portion of the transverse colon results in the movement of colonic content toward the rectum. At times, luminal material travels rather slowly. However, it can move rapidly all the way to the rectum if mass propulsion occurs. When the semi-dried fecal material reaches the rectum, it may distend the rectum sufficiently to initiate the defecation reflex. If defecation is voluntarily suppressed, the fecal mass is stored or moved back toward the sigmoid colon. Retrograde movement of feces occurs because the slow wave frequency (and contractile activity) in the rectum is higher than in the sigmoid colon.

The transit of chyme in the large intestine is expressed in terms of days rather than hours. On a Western diet, three to four days are required for a given bolus of material to travel from the ileocecal junction to the rectum. The fiber content of the diet is a major determinant of colonic transit time (Fig. 8–8). This fact is demonstrated by the reduction in transit time (4 days to 2 days) when a large amount of bran (fiber) is added to the diet.

DEFECATION

Anatomic Considerations

The rectum and anus are particularly well suited for the controlled elimination of feces. The rectal mucosa contains crypts, which are deeper than those of the rest of the colon and are almost exclusively populated by goblet cells. The mucous secretion produced by these cells presumably lubricates the rectal surface and eases the passage of semi-solid stools. The surface epithelium changes progressively from columnar epithelia to a stratified squamous epithelium, which, at the level of the anal orifice, becomes epidermis. The exit of fecal material is controlled by two sphincters encircling the anal canal. The circular smooth muscle of the anal canal is three to four times thicker than that in the remainder of the colon and forms the internal anal sphincter. The longitudinal muscle layer becomes thinner over the internal sphincter and inserts

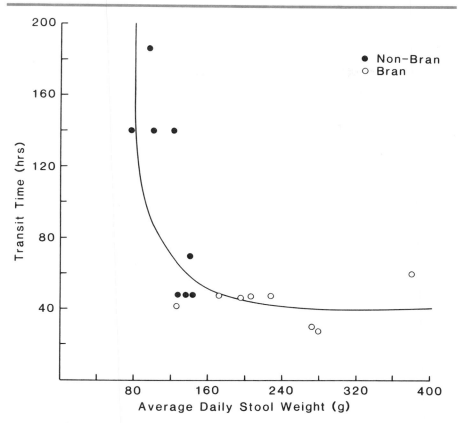

FIGURE 8–8.   The effect of dietary fiber on colonic transit time and stool weight. (From Connell, A.M. *In* Reilly, R.W., and Kirsner, J.B. (eds.): Fiber Deficiency and Colonic Disorders. New York, Plenum Publishing Corp., 1975, p. 82.)

into adjacent connective tissue. The internal anal sphincter is surrounded by several bundles of striated muscle, which form the external anal sphincter.

INNERVATION OF INTERNAL AND EXTERNAL ANAL SPHINCTERS

The internal anal sphincter is innervated by the autonomic nervous system. The parasympathetic supply is via the pelvic nerves, whereas sympathetic fibers are supplied by the hypogastric nerves. Activation of the parasympathetic nerves results in relaxation of the internal anal sphincter, a response mediated by the inhibitory neurons of the myenteric plexus. Sympathetic discharge tends to constrict the internal sphincter by activating α-adrenergic receptors on the smooth muscle.

The external anal sphincter, composed of striated muscle, receives somatic innervation via the pudendal nerves. The innervation of the external sphincter

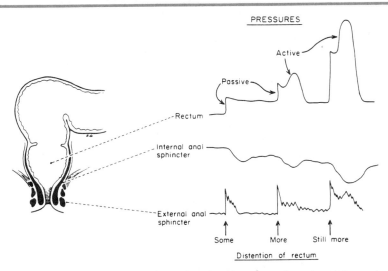

FIGURE 8–9. Response of the rectum and anal sphincters to distention of the rectum. Mild distention of the rectum stretches its walls and causes a passive increase in pressure. Further distention reinforces the passive increases in pressure by stimulating contraction of the rectal walls. Each increment in rectal pressure is accompanied by a decrease in pressure at the internal sphincter and an increase in pressure at the external sphincter. (From Davenport, H.W.: Physiology of the Digestive Tract, 4th ed. Chicago, Year Book Medical Publishers, 1977, p. 79.)

is excitatory, and the sphincter can be paralyzed by cutting the pudendal nerves. Like skeletal muscle, the external sphincter is primarily under voluntary control.

Reflex Activity of the Anal Sphincters

Both the internal and external anal sphincters are tonically constricted. However, the reflex responses of the two sphincters to rectal distention are different and provide the basis for the defecation reflex (Fig. 8–9). Mild distention of the rectum results in a passive increase in rectal pressure. If the distention pressure is great enough, the passive increase in pressure is reinforced by an active contraction of the rectal muscles. The internal sphincter relaxes as the rectum is distended, an event mediated by intrinsic nerves. The external sphincter contracts in response to rectal distention. The contraction is mediated through an extrinsic somatic reflex activated by stretch receptors in the rectum.

Continence

As feces enters the rectum, either slowly during the interdigestive period or as a result of a mass propulsive wave after a meal, the rectal lumen distends. If the volume of the fecal mass is sufficiently large, rectal contractions ensue, and the urge to defecate is felt. Although the internal anal sphincter relaxes in response to rectal distention, the external sphincter contracts (Fig. 8–9). If the urge to defecate is opposed by voluntary contraction of the extenal anal sphincter, the rectal receptors eventually adapt, and the internal sphincter regains its tone. The rectum accommodates the fecal mass or propels it toward the sigmoid colon, and the urge to defecate subsides. This ability of the individual to override the urge to defecate by voluntary control of the external sphincters is referred to as continence.

Act of Defecation

If the rectum is appropriately distended at a convenient time either by the entrance of feces into the rectum or a voluntary increase in abdominal pressure, the defecation reflex will be voluntarily reinforced. The internal sphincter will relax, but the external sphincter will only transiently constrict owing to voluntary removal of excitatory input to this sphincter. When both sphincters are relaxed, the increased rectal pressure will move the stool through the anal orifice. This basic defecation reflex is reinforced by extrinsic reflexes, which are mediated by the pelvic nerves. Activation of these nerves by rectal receptors causes contractions of the descending and sigmoid colon and enhances the intrinsic inhibitory influence on the internal anal sphincter. Increased pelvic nerve activity also releases VIP which, in turn, increases mucus secretion in the distal colon to facilitate the movement of feces. This extrinsic parasympathetic reflex can actually result in emptying of the descending and sigmoid colon as well as the rectum. The sympathetic nerves do not contribute significantly to the act of defecation.

Evacuation of the rectum is assisted by voluntary acts such as the Valsalva maneuver and by assuming a squatting position. The Valsalva maneuver consists of a forced expiration against a closed glottis, which increases intra-abdominal pressure. The increase in abdominal pressure forces the pelvic floor downward, straightening the anorectal angle and thereby reducing the resistance to the movement of feces. Flexion of the hips while assuming the squatting position also helps in aligning the anorectal angle.

Most people defecate once a day. However, defecation frequencies of two per day or one every two days are within the normal range. The weight of the stool can vary considerably from one individual to another and from one bowel movement to another, determined largely by the fiber content of the diet (Fig. 8–8). The fecal water content, however, remains relatively constant. The amount of solids contained in the stool largely determines stool weight. Seventy per cent of the total solids in stools consist of bacteria and fiber. There do not appear to be any differences between healthy males and females with regard to size, volume, and frequency of stools.

COLONIC CIRCULATION

Resting colonic blood flow in the adult human is approximately 250 ml per minute, which accounts for 5 per cent of cardiac output. Blood flows as large as 1500 ml per minute (30 per cent of resting cardiac output) have been measured in the colon of patients with ulcerative colitis. In humans, colonic blood flow (per unit mass of tissue) is approximately 40 per cent and 60 per cent of blood flow values measured in jejunum and ileum, respectively. The proximal colon receives a greater share of blood flow than the more distal portion.

Blood flow within the colon is unevenly distributed between the mucosa-submucosa (65 per cent) and muscularis (35 per cent) layers, reflecting the different demands of the tissue layers for oxygen and other nutrients. Sympathetic nerve stimulation reduces total colonic blood flow while redistributing flow to the mucosa-submucosa layers, i.e., the vasoconstriction is more pronounced in the muscle layers. Pelvic (parasympathetic) nerve stimulation produces a biphasic (intense transient hyperemia followed by a smaller rhythmic hyperemia) increase in colonic blood flow, with the initial hyperemia confined to the superficial mucosal layer. The initial hyperemia is believed to be mediated by vasoactive intestinal polypeptide, which is released as a neurotransmitter from terminal fibers of the pelvic nerve. The sustained rhythmic hyperemia induced by parasympathetic activation is blocked by atropine.

Blood flow to the colon increases approximately 45 minutes following a meal. The postprandial hyperemia is confined to the mucosal layer, and the mechanism(s) mediating the vascular response have not been characterized. The volatile short-chain fatty acids produced by bacterial degradation of carbohydrates may mediate the hyperemia, since they increase blood flow when instilled into the lumen of the colon. The postprandial hyperemia may also involve a local nervous reflex.

In contrast to the small intestine, net water absorption in the colon does not produce a rise in lymph flow. The absorbed fluid is removed from the colonic interstitium exclusively by the blood capillaries. The relative contributions of the blood and lymph microcirculations in transporting absorbed fluid is consistent with the distribution of these vessels in the colon. The initial lymphatics in the colonic mucosa are of a much smaller caliber than the lacteals of the small intestine, and they are located some 300 μm from the absorptive epithelium (the lacteals of the small intestine are about 50 μm from the enterocytes). Furthermore, the fenestrated capillaries of the colonic mucosa are much closer to the absorptive cells (1 μm) than their counterparts in the small intestine (2 μm), which is advantageous for the removal of absorbed fluid via the capillaries.

COLONIC PAIN

As in the small intestine, colonic pain arises from distention and stretching of the bowel wall. Nerve fibers conveying this sensation are found in the muscle layer. The pain is generally referred to the hypogastrium. Rectal pain is felt posteriorly, over the sacrum.

CLINICAL CORRELATIONS

The colon is prone to many diseases, such as carcinoma and ulcerative colitis, a chronic inflammatory disease of unknown cause. In addition, a huge number of patients consult their doctors regarding symptoms such as colonic pain, constipation, and diarrhea; in some instances, these may reflect some serious organic disease but, in others, they result from dysfunction of a colon which is structurally normal.

The osmotic action of certain luminal constituents opposes normal water and electrolyte absorption from the bowel lumen. Osmotic laxatives such as magnesium sulfate act in this way in both small intestine and colon. Unabsorbed lactose in subjects who are deficient in the brush border enzyme lactase holds water in the lumen of the small intestine (see Fig. 7–15). However, in the colon, bacteria metabolize the lactose to CO_2, H_2, and water. When fat is malabsorbed in the small intestine, fatty acids enter the colon and bacteria hydroxylate them to compounds, such as 10-hydroxystearic acid, which are powerful secretagogues in the colon; thus steatorrhea is accompanied by increased stool water.

Bile acids are normally conserved in the enterohepatic circulation. Approximately 10 per cent of the bile acid pool ($\sim$ 300 mg) passes daily into the colon. Bacteria modify these bile acids. A major stool bile acid is deoxycholic acid, produced by dehydroxylation and deconjugation of glyco- or taurocholic acid. This bile acid, like the hydroxy-fatty acids, is a secretagogue in the colon. The term "cholerrheic enteropathy" has been applied to the situation in which excessive amounts of bile acids enter the colon and cause diarrhea as the result of terminal ileal disease or resection. Interestingly, in the rare cases of congenital bile salt deficiency, intractable constipation is a prominent feature; this deficiency suggests that bile salts may normally regulate the consistency of the stool. Irritant purgatives such as senna are also secretagogues in the colon.

In ulcerative colitis involving a large area of the colon, diarrhea is the result of extensive mucosal inflammation and edema. In this situation, protein-rich fluid exudes from the mucosa. Frank bleeding from the mucosa is also common.

If the diet is poor in nonabsorbable residue, as Western Hemisphere diets tend to be, there is comparatively little solid matter in the ileal effluent. Water absorption by the colon produces small, hard, pellety stools. Colonic smooth muscle has difficulty in propelling the material, and constipation is likely to result. Like other hollow organs with smooth muscle in the wall, the colon responds to distention with high residue material by contraction. Thus, in Third

World countries where the diet is high in residue, the transit time of fecal material through the colon is much faster than in North America. Dietary fiber (the nonabsorbable residue) holds water like a sponge and helps to give the stool a soft consistency for easy evacuation. Rather than change their eating habits to include more roughage, many North Americans would prefer to take special fiber preparations (as pills, grains, or powder), which are commercially available.

In some patients, constipation is the result of a generalized depression of smooth muscle activity in the body. A good example of this generalized depression is the constipation of pregnancy, where high circulating levels of progesterone depress the tone of visceral smooth muscle.

REFERENCES

Binder, H.J.: Absorption and secretion of water and electrolytes by small and large intestine. In Sleisenger, M.H., and Fordtran, J.S. (eds.): Gastrointestinal Disease: Pathophysiology, Diagnosis, Management, 3rd ed. Philadelphia, W.B. Saunders Co., 1983, pp. 811–827.

Binder, H.J.: Colonic secretion. In Johnson, L.R. (ed.): Physiology of the Gastrointestinal Tract. New York, Raven Press, 1981, pp. 1003–1015.

Christensen, J.: Motility of the colon. In Johnson, L.R. (ed.): Physiology of the Gastrointestinal Tract. New York, Raven Press, 1981, pp. 445–471.

Cohen, S., and Snape, W.J.: Movement of the small and large intestine. In Sleisenger, M.H., and Fordtran, J.S. (eds.): Gastrointestinal Disease: Pathophysiology, Diagnosis, Management, 3rd ed. Philadelphia, W.B. Saunders Co., 1983, pp. 859–873.

Devroede, G.: Storage and propulsion along the large intestine. In Bustos-Fernandez, L. (ed.): Colon Structure and Function. New York, Plenum Medical Book Co., 1983, pp. 121–139.

Haubrich, W.S.: Anatomy of the colon. In Bockus, H.L. (ed.): Gastroenterology, Vol. 2. Philadelphia, W.B. Saunders Co., 1976, pp. 595–618.

Jewell, D.P., and Selby, W.S.: Immunology of the colon. In Bustos-Fernandez, L. (ed.): Colon Structure and Function. New York, Plenum Medical Book Co., 1983, pp. 79–101.

Kerlin, P., and Phillips, S.: Absorption and secretion of electrolytes by the human colon. In Bustos-Fernandez, L. (ed.): Colon Structure and Function. New York, Plenum Medical Book Co., 1983, pp. 17–37.

Kvietys, P.R., and Granger, D.N.: Physiology, pharmacology and pathology of the colonic circulation. In Shepherd, A.P., and Granger, D.N. (eds.): Physiology of the Intestinal Circulation. New York, Raven Press, 1984, pp. 131–143.

Levitt, M.D., Bond, J.H., and Levitt, D.G.: Gastrointestinal gas. In Johnson, L.R. (ed.): Physiology of the Gastrointestinal Tract. New York, Raven Press, 1981, pp. 1301–1316.

Menge, H., and Robinson, J.W.L.: Colonic adaptation. In Bustos-Fernandez, L. (ed.): Colon Structure and Function. New York, Plenum Medical Book Co., 1983, pp. 253–273.

Patton, J.S.: Gastrointestinal lipid digestion. In Johnson, L.R. (ed.): Physiology of the Gastrointestinal Tract. New York, Raven Press, 1981, pp. 1124–1141.

Polak, J.M., Bishop, A.E., and Bloom, S.R.: The regulatory peptides of the colon. In Bustos-Fernandez, L. (ed.): Colon Structure and Function. New York, Plenum Medical Book Co., 1983, pp. 167–186.

Roman, C., and Gonella, J.: Extrinsic control of digestive tract motility. In Johnson, L.R. (ed.): Physiology of the Gastrointestinal Tract. New York, Raven Press, 1981, pp. 289–333.

Schultz, S.G.: Ion transport by mammalian large intestine. In Johnson, L.R. (ed.): Physiology of the Gastrointestinal Tract. New York, Raven Press, 1981, pp. 991–1004.

Simon, G.L., and Gorbach, S.L.: Bacteriology of the colon. In Bustos-Fernandez, L. (ed.): Colon Structure and Function. New York, Plenum Medical Book Co., 1983, pp. 103–116.

Sodeman, W.A., and Watson, D.W.: The large intestine. *In* Sodeman, W.A., and Sodeman, T.M. (eds.): Pathologic Physiology: Mechanisms of Disease. Philadelphia, W.B. Saunders Co., 1974, pp. 767–789.

Trier, J.S., Krone, C.L., and Sleisenger, M.H.: Anatomy, embryology and developmental abnormalities of the small intestine and colon. *In* Sleisenger, M.H., and Fordtran, J.S. (eds.): Gastrointestinal Disease: Pathophysiology, Diagnosis, Management, 3rd ed. Philadelphia, W.B. Saunders Co., 1983, pp. 780–811.

In the preceding chapters, particular emphasis was placed on the physiologic functions of individual organs composing the digestive system. While all of the digestive organs make a significant contribution to the overall assimilation of foodstuffs, the onset and magnitude of their contribution(s) vary considerably. The objective of this chapter is to provide a qualitative overview of how the individual organs of this system interact in a concerted fashion to efficiently process a meal. This process will be described in terms of the traditional division of the overall response to a meal, i.e., the cephalic, gastric, and intestinal phases.

The digestive system of man is continuously active. However, approximately three times a day the system is challenged by ingestion of meals, and the response of the system is characterized by periods of intense activity. Because the composition of meals varies, the intensity and character of the responses are similarly variable. The specific characteristics of a meal that are important in this regard are its appeal, size, consistency (proportion of solid and liquid), tonicity, and the relative proportion of the three major nutrients (carbohydrates, lipids, and protein). The responses to a meal described in the foregoing discussion relate to an appetizing meal containing a balanced mixture of the three major nutrients. The meal is taken along with liberal amounts of fluid, resulting in an isotonic mixture entering the stomach.

9

INTEGRATED RESPONSE OF THE DIGESTIVE SYSTEM TO A MEAL

INTERDIGESTIVE PERIOD

Twelve to fifteen hours per day are spent in the interdigestive period, which is characterized by a low basal level of motor, secretory, and digestive activity (Fig. 9–1). This basal activity can be attributed to low levels of parasympathetic drive and circulating gastrointestinal hormones. During this period, there is continuous exfoliation and regeneration of the mucosal epithelium. Also, at this time, the endocrine and exocrine cells are replenishing their depleted stores of hormones and digestive enzymes.

The salivary glands are secreting saliva at a basal rate to moisten the oral

INTERDIGESTIVE PERIOD

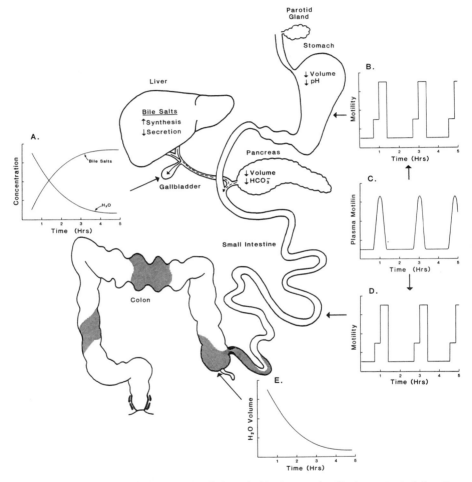

FIGURE 9–1. The interdigestive period. This period is characterized by low output of digestive secretions and the migrating motility complex (MMC). The contractile patterns in the stomach (*B*) and intestine (*D*) are correlated to the plasma concentration of motilin (*C*). Water and electrolytes are being absorbed in the gallbladder (*A*) and cecum (*E*).

mucosa and prevent bacterial overgrowth. The esophageal sphincters (upper and lower) are constricted, and the esophagus is collapsed. The intraesophageal pressure is cycling with respiration. This pattern is interrupted intermittently by swallowing (primary peristaltic waves); about half of all swallows occur during the interdigestive period. If gastroesophageal reflux occurs (e.g., while reclining), secondary peristaltic waves clear the esophagus.

Gastric juice is produced at a low level so that the stomach contains a low volume of highly acidic fluid. The low intragastric pH is due to the absence of food, which acts as a buffer. Reduced vagal drive directly suppresses acid secretion by the parietal cells and indirectly decreases acid output by reduced stimulation of gastrin release from the antrum. The low intragastric pH further suppresses acid production by directly inhibiting gastrin release. Gastric motor activity is characterized by oscillations between periods of quiescence and bursts of activity, with cycles occurring every one to two hours. This pattern of motor activity (migrating motility complex) is dictated by circulating levels of motilin (Fig. 9–1). The acidic fluid containing cellular debris is gradually emptied from the stomach through a partially closed pylorus.

The pancreas is producing a low bicarbonate, low enzyme juice at a minimal rate, presumably owing to a low activity of its neural (vagal) and humoral (secretin and cholecystokinin) stimulants. The pancreatic juice periodically spurts into the duodenal lumen because of intermittent relaxation of the sphincter of Oddi. The alkaline pancreatic juice buffers the small amount of acidic gastric juice entering the duodenum.

During the interdigestive period, the concentration of bile salts in portal venous blood is low; therefore, the rate of hepatic bile salt synthesis is high and the rate of secretion is low. Since the sphincter of Oddi is closed (with brief periods of relaxation), bile flow is preferentially diverted to the gallbladder. Within the gallbladder water is absorbed, producing a more concentrated bile. Most of the total bile salt pool is located in the gallbladder at this time.

The small bowel is virtually empty during the interdigestive period; only a small volume of residue remains in the terminal ileum. The motor activity of the small bowel is characterized by periodic (1 to 2 hrs) bursts of contractions that are caused by corresponding increases in circulating motilin. The migrating motility complex acts as a "housekeeper" which prevents bacterial overgrowth. In contrast to the small bowel, the colon contains a considerable amount of food residue. In the proximal colon, haustral shuttling mixes the watery mass and continually exposes it to the mucosal surface, where water and electrolytes are efficiently absorbed. The distal colon is either empty or is storing semisolid feces.

DIGESTIVE PERIOD

The Cephalic Phase

Anticipation of a familiar and appetizing meal activates central parasympathetic efferents. When the individual is then presented with the meal, the

DIGESTIVE PERIOD: CEPHALIC PHASE

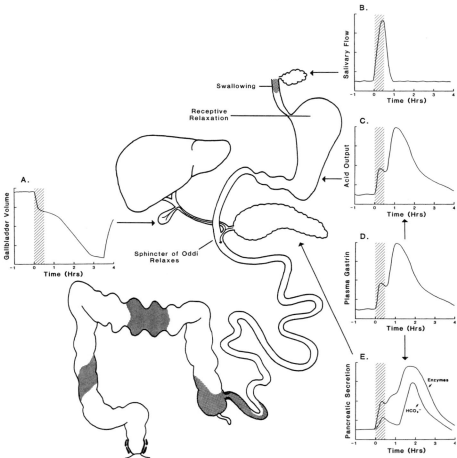

FIGURE 9–2. The cephalic phase of digestion. This period is characterized by an activated parasympathetic system and a small rise in plasma gastrin (D). These neurohumoral factors increase salivary (B), gastric (C), and pancreatic (E) secretions. The gallbladder contracts (A) and the sphincter of Oddi relaxes.

parasympathetic component of the autonomic nervous system is further activated by afferent information (sight and smell) from the sense organs. As eating commences, gustatory afferents reinforce the enhanced parasympathetic drive. The resulting efferent activity, which is mainly vagal, stimulates secretion by digestive glands, thereby preparing the gastrointestinal tract for the incoming food. This entire process is termed the cephalic phase (Fig. 9–2).

Salivary secretion increases about sixfold during the cephalic phase. The increased salivary flow provides the required lubrication for comfortable and efficient mastication and deglutition. Food in the mouth initiates the swallowing reflex, which involves relaxation of the upper esophageal sphincter and peristaltic propulsion of the food bolus toward the stomach. The lower esophageal sphincter relaxes, allowing the bolus to pass into the stomach. When liquids are ingested, multiple swallows are involved, and gravity plays an important role in esophageal transport.

As soon as swallowing occurs, adaptive relaxation of the gastric fundus begins, allowing the stomach to fill with a minimal rise in pressure. Gastric secretion increases, the result of direct vagal action (acetylcholine) and, more importantly, vagal release of gastrin. The increased acid secretion during the cephalic phase accounts for about 30 per cent of the maximal response to a meal. Unlike the gastric secretory response, pancreatic cephalic secretion is primarily driven by direct vagal action, producing a low volume, enzyme-rich juice. The increased circulating levels of gastrin serve to augment the vagal effect. Relaxation of the sphincter of Oddi (also mediated by the vagus) allows the pancreatic juice to enter the duodenum. The relaxed sphincter, coupled to vagally induced gallbladder contraction, permits up to 30 per cent of stored bile to be emptied into the gut. Hepatic bile salt synthesis and secretion rates are comparable to those observed in the interdigestive period.

The interdigestive pattern of motor activity in the small and large intestine is minimally influenced by the cephalic phase.

The enhanced secretory activity of the salivary, gastric, and pancreatic glands is associated with increased metabolic demands that are met by corresponding increases in blood flow. In addition, microvascular adjustments lead to enhanced capillary filtration, thereby providing the fluid for secretion.

The Gastric Phase

The gastric phase can be defined as that period of time during which food is in the stomach (Fig. 9–3). Since food enters the stomach at the start of a meal there is no clear demarcation between the cephalic and gastric phases. Nonetheless, there are specific events, related to digestive function, that result from the presence of food in the stomach. In general, the parasympathetic influence is waning while gastrin is becoming a more dominant factor at this stage.

A feature of the waning parasympathetic influence of the cephalic phase is the gradual decline of salivary flow toward the basal level. Swallowing and associated esophageal peristaltic activity continues as long as the meal is being ingested. Food continues to enter the stomach, causing further distention with little rise in intragastric pressure. Gastric distention stimulates stretch receptors, initiating a vago-vagal reflex, which maintains parietal cell secretion. The major stimulus of parietal cell secretion in this phase is antral gastrin released by the products of protein digestion. The pH of gastric contents rises (from about 1 to about 4) as a result of the buffering action of the food. This releases the inhibition of gastrin release exerted by low antral pH. Pepsin catalyzes

DIGESTIVE PERIOD: GASTRIC PHASE

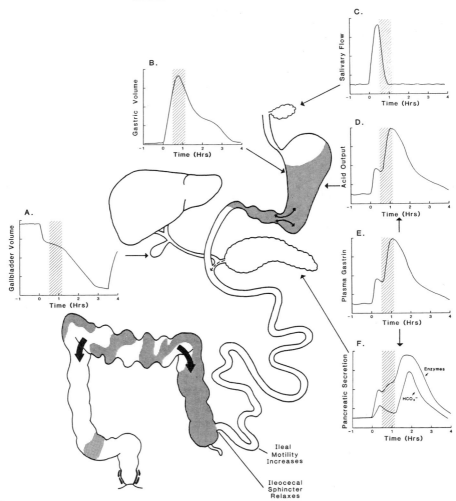

FIGURE 9–3. The gastric phase of digestion. This period is characterized by a decreased parasympathetic drive and a further increase in plasma gastrin (*E*). Salivary secretion returns toward the basal level (*C*), whereas gastric (*D*) and pancreatic (*F*) secretions are further augmented. Gastric volume increases rapidly and subsequently declines as it empties (*B*). The gallbladder continues to empty (*A*). Motor reflexes from the stomach initiate ileal and colonic contractions; chyme moves into the cecum where it is mixed.

protein hydrolysis, and a limited amount of lipolysis occurs by lingual lipase. Highly lipid-soluble substances such as ethanol and some fatty acids are absorbed in the stomach. Vigorous antral contractions, which generate high lumen pressures, reduce particle size and form a coarse emulsion of the gastric content. Gastric emptying proceeds at a rate dictated by the consistency of chyme, i.e., liquids at a greater rate than digestible solids, and digestible solids at a greater rate than nondigestible solids.

Despite the reduced vagal activity, the rate of pancreatic secretion (rich in enzymes) is sustained owing to increased circulating levels of gastrin. The gallbladder continues to empty during the gastric phase but at a slower rate because of reduced parasympathetic drive.

The rise in circulating gastrin levels initiates the gastroileal reflex; peristaltic activity increases in the terminal ileum, the ileocecal sphincter relaxes, the chyme from a previous meal is propelled into the cecum. Gastrin also initiates the gastrocolic reflex, which increases haustral shuttling (cecum) and propulsive activity (transverse colon).

Blood flow to the digestive system remains elevated during the gastric phase; however, the hyperemia in the salivary gland is waning while gastric mucosal blood flow rises to a higher level.

The Intestinal Phase

The intestinal phase can be defined as that period of time in which chyme is present in the small intestine. Since chyme is emptied from the stomach over a long period of time there is considerable overlap between the gastric and intestinal phases. Events that occur exclusively during the intestinal phase are release of intestinal hormones (CCK, secretin) and the digestion and absorption of all three classes of nutrients.

EARLY PERIOD

Feedback inhibition of secretory and motor activity of the stomach occurs during the early intestinal phase (Fig. 9–4). Included in this response is a progressive reduction in the rate of gastric emptying, which is mediated by humoral and neural mechanisms. The luminal factors responsible for inhibition of gastric emptying are duodenal acidity (secretin), lipids (CCK), distention or irritation (vago-vagal reflex), and hypertonicity. As a result of the strong inhibition exerted by lipids in the duodenum, a fatty meal may remain in the stomach for as long as three hours. Inasmuch as large food particles must be further reduced in size before passing the pylorus, the antral mill continues to churn (retroperistalsis). Gastric acid secretion begins to fall during the intestinal phase owing to a falling pH in the lumen of both the stomach and duodenum. The loss of food (buffer) from the stomach as it empties acidifies the antrum, which in turn suppresses the release of gastrin. Duodenal acidity stimulates secretin release, which further depresses parietal cell acid output.

DIGESTIVE PERIOD: EARLY INTESTINAL PHASE

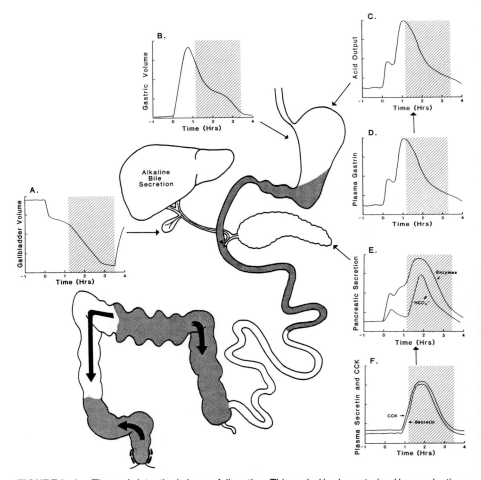

FIGURE 9–4.   The early intestinal phase of digestion. This period is characterized by a reduction in plasma gastrin levels (*D*) and a concomitant rise in plasma levels of secretin and CCK (*F*). The stomach continues to slowly empty its contents (*B*), while acid output falls dramatically (*C*). The pancreas elaborates an enzyme- and bicarbonate-rich secretion (*E*). There is intense contraction of the gallbladder (*A*). The motor pattern in the small bowel shifts from the MMC to irregular segmental and propulsive contractions, which mix the chyme with digestive secretions. Colonic motility includes patterns such as mass movements and retropulsion.

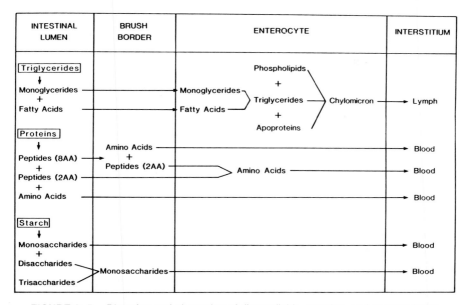

FIGURE 9–5. Digestion and absorption of dietary lipids, proteins, and carbohydrates.

The pancreatic secretory response reaches its maximum level during the early intestinal phase. The pancreatic juice is rich in both bicarbonate and enzymes, which neutralizes acidic chyme and achieves optimum hydrolysis of nutrients. The secretory response is mediated by secretin and CCK, which potentiate each other's action. The intestinal hormones are released in response to duodenal acidity (secretin) and the hydrolytic products of lipid and protein digestion (CCK).

As a result of cholecystokinin release, there is intense contraction of the gallbladder and concomitant relaxation of the sphincter of Oddi, so that 80 per cent of the interdigestive gallbladder volume is emptied into the duodenum. Secretin stimulates the production of a bicarbonate-rich biliary secretion.

Entrance of food into the small intestine disrupts the interdigestive motor pattern (MMC) and initiates mixing (segmentation) and propulsive (peristalsis) contractions. The digestive pattern of motility promotes digestion of nutrients in the lumen (Fig. 9–5). The lipolytic enzymes of pancreatic juice hydrolyze triglycerides to monoglycerides and fatty acids. These products are solubilized in bile salt micelles, in which they are delivered to the enterocyte. Once they passively diffuse into the cell, the monoglycerides and fatty acids are used to form triglycerides, which are subsequently incorporated into chylomicrons. The chylomicrons leave the enterocyte and gain access to the systemic circulation via the lymphatics. The complement of pancreatic proteases hydrolyzes dietary proteins to small peptides and amino acids. Amino acids are actively transported into the enterocyte. The larger peptides (> 3 amino acids) are hydrolyzed by enzymes in the brush border to di- and tripeptides, which are actively transported into the cell and subsequently hydrolyzed to amino acids. The amino acids in the cell then diffuse into portal venous blood. Pancreatic amylase cleaves starch to a mixture of small oligosaccharides and glucose. The oligosaccharides are further hydrolyzed by brush border enzymes to glucose. The glucose is actively transported into the enterocyte and then diffuses into the portal vein.

In the early intestinal phase the elevated levels of CCK and gastrin initiate haustral and propulsive movements in the colon. Often, this results in a "mass movement" of fecal material from the distal transverse colon to as far as the rectum. Distention of the rectum will initiate the defecation reflex; the internal anal sphincter relaxes and the external anal sphincter transiently constricts. If the urge to defecate is voluntarily suppressed the rectum adapts and the internal sphincter regains its tone. The fecal material will be stored or retropulsed into the sigmoid colon.

Blood flow to the digestive system rises to a greater level during the early intestinal phase, primarily owing to a further increase in pancreatic blood flow and an intense hyperemia in the mucosal layer of the small bowel. However, gastric mucosal blood flow begins to decline because of inhibition of acid secretion.

LATE PERIOD

When the upper small intestine is virtually empty owing to absorption of water, electrolytes, and nutrients, the stimuli for hormone release from the duodenum and jejunum have been removed. Thus, the rates of gastric and pancreatic secretions gradually fall toward interdigestive levels (Fig. 9–6). In the terminal ileum, bile salts are actively reabsorbed, producing a rise in their portal venous blood concentration. This suppresses liver synthesis of bile salts while stimulating hepatic bile salt secretion. It is estimated that a meal results in two to three enterohepatic cycles of the bile salt pool. As a result of enhanced bile flow into the biliary tract and closure of the sphincter of Oddi, the gallbladder slowly begins to fill with hepatic bile.

In the late intestinal phase, gastric and small intestinal motor activities shift from the irregular digestive pattern to the cyclic interdigestive pattern (the migrating motility complex). Chyme continues to move into the cecum. Colonic segmental and propulsive activity results in further accumulation of fecal material in the rectum. Subsequent rectal distention will elicit the defecation reflex, which, if not opposed voluntarily, will result in passage of stool.

EXAGGERATED PHYSIOLOGIC RESPONSES TO FEEDING

In response to a meal, some individuals experience symptoms which result from exaggerated physiologic responses to stimulation of the gastrointestinal

DIGESTIVE PERIOD: LATE INTESTINAL PHASE

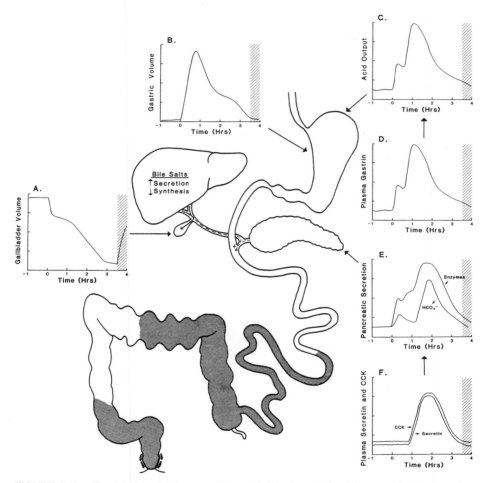

FIGURE 9–6. The late intestinal phase. This period is characterized by a gradual return of the intestinal hormones (secretin and CCK) to their interdigestive plasma levels (*D, F*). Gastric (*C*) and pancreatic (*E*) secretion rates and gastric volume (*B*) fall toward their basal levels. Bile salts, absorbed from the terminal ileum, stimulate hepatic bile salt secretion and inhibit bile salt synthesis. The gallbladder slowly fills with hepatic bile (*A*). When the rectum distends sufficiently, the urge to defecate is felt and the stool is passed.

tract. These include a marked gastrocolic reflex with a call to stool during eating, a phenomenon commonly observed in the newborn, in whom a bowel movement often accompanies feeding. In some individuals, intense stimulation of gustatory receptors (e.g., with highly spiced food) leads to marked facial vasodilatation (flushing), nasal secretion, and lacrimation. The exaggerated gustatory effects are consistent with an enhanced parasympathetic response.

The dumping syndrome, a problem which often arises after gastric surgery, may also occur in the normal individual whose rate of gastric emptying is fast. In this condition, the arrival of a hyperosmotic load in the upper small intestine results in the movement of water from the circulation, across the mucosa, and into the gut lumen. Contraction of intravascular volume leads to symptoms such as dizziness, tachycardia, and a pounding pulse 15 to 30 minutes after eating. It has been proposed that these symptoms may also arise from the release of peptides or other biologically active substances from the intestine. A late dumping syndrome, occurring about 1.5 to 2 hours after eating and characterized by weakness, sweating, and tachycardia is thought to be a result of hypoglycemia associated with excessive release of insulin in the postprandial period.

INDEX

Letters in *italics* refer to illustrations; letters followed by (t) refer to tables.